Joining the Club

To Millie
A special club member

Lillie Shockney

Joining the Club

The Reality of Breast Cancer

Lillie Shockney

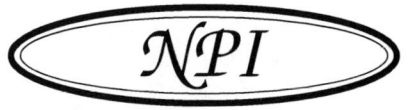

Northwest Publishing, Inc,
Salt Lake City, Utah

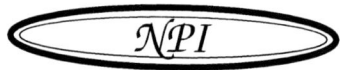

All rights reserved
Copyright © 1995 Northwest Publishing, Inc,

Reproduction in any manner, in whole or in part,
in English or in other languages, or otherwise
without written permission of the publisher is prohibited.

For information address: Northwest Publishing, Inc.,
6906 South 300 West, Salt Lake City, Utah 84047
BCC 12.13.94

PRINTING HISTORY
First Printing 1995

ISBN 1-56901-524-4

NPI books are published by Northwest Publishing, Inc,
6906 South 300 West, Salt Lake City, Utah 84047
The name "NPI" and the "NPI" logo are trademarks belonging to
Northwest Publishing, Incorporated

PRINTED IN THE UNITED STATES OF AMERICA
10 9 8 7 6 5 4 3 2 1

This book is dedicated to:

My husband, Al, for showing me that
his love for me is eternal.

My daughter, Laura, for sharing with me the wisdom and
humor that a loving child can provide
in a crisis situation.

My parents, who provided me their continued love and
support and reaffirmed my belief of "once
a parent, always a parent."

The late John Cross for being my guardian angel.

My surgeon, Charlie Yeo, for providing me the surgical
skills and professional compassion I needed
to become a breast cancer survivor.

Chapter 1

I guess it is best that we don't know what our future holds in store for us, because if we did, we'd convince ourselves that we'd rather not go through certain experiences—sometimes even if the end result was to be positive. I once read on a bumper sticker the definition of an experience:

*An experience is what you get when you
don't get what you want.*

For those of us who have had breast cancer, still have breast cancer, or love someone with such a diagnosis, we are among those who have had "an experience."

I've had the unique opportunity to experience breast cancer from three different perspectives: as a teenager who watched the impact a diagnosis of breast cancer had on someone I loved and feared losing; as a registered nurse who cared for women treated for this disease; and as a woman who became a mastectomy patient.

This book is a story about these three experiences and how they have affected my life and that of my family. I will be very candid with you because I feel that it's important for you to be given an opportunity to gain a sense of how this disease may affect you. If you are a woman who has been diagnosed with breast cancer or fear being diagnosed in the future, I hope you find information about my experience helpful emotionally, physically, and spiritually. If you are a nurse or other health care professional involved in the care and treatment of women with breast cancer, I hope you feel a sense of what it's like to be on the receiving end of such care. After all, with one in nine women being diagnosed with breast cancer, you could be in my shoes (or bra) one day.

I have also provided resource information for breast cancer patients, families, and friends who are in need of access to medical information, emotional support, or other resources. This is my story…

Born and reared on a dairy farm outside of Chestertown, Maryland, I had a lot of opportunities for experiences with accidental mishaps, which is why my parents always made sure that I had a tetanus shot every spring. I used to get really mad at them about my having to get that shot. You see, my brother got to go to camp every summer and as part of the camp regulations he had to get a tetanus shot. I, on the other hand, didn't get to go to camp but they made me get a tetanus shot anyway. Now, as an adult, I can see that they were using good judgment and saving themselves a repeat trip back to the doctor's office that was nearly an hour away from the farm where we lived, because before the summer was out, I would have needed a tetanus shot anyway. I also think that this is probably the reason why they never let me go to camp either—I was an accident looking for a place to happen! Every year I'd ask, "Can I go to camp with Robert?" and every year the answer would be, "You are not old enough to go to camp." Then one year when I asked again my ritualistic annual question, "Can I go to camp?" The response was different. They said, "Camp? Why, you are too *old* to go to camp." (Gee, I guess my opportunity to "experience" camp would have been the *winter* of my eleventh year of life . . .) So as you can probably surmise, whenever I am mad at my folks now that I am an adult, I usually throw in a zinger like, "And by the way, you never let me go to camp, either!" That way they know that I still think I should have had the experience to injure myself in a fun location and not just have my medical mishaps on the farm.

Whether I felt the need to have medical expertise to know how to take care of myself or if it was due to my impulse to take care of other people, it is still a mystery to me as to what the driving force was that steered me toward a career in nursing. I'd like to believe that it was (and still is) the compassionate side of me but certainly part of my brain might have been reaching back into my childhood and wanted to make absolutely sure that all of those trips to the doctor's office (and all of those tetanus and penicillin shots) were truly necessary. From the time I was a youngster I wanted to be a nurse.

When I had just begun my teenage years, a couple moved to a home not very far from our farm. The wife of the couple took a liking to me as well as to my mom. Though she was at least ten years older than my mother, Miss Bertha (as I chose to call her) had the spirit of a child. I was basically a loner in school, partly because I was known as a bookworm and partly because I didn't live near other children. Our farm was nine miles from the next town and more than one mile from another family with children. So, despite the fact that Miss Bertha was old enough to be my mother (or possibly even my grandmother), she became a best friend to me. She enjoyed having me over and liked to practice cheerleading routines with me. She also taught me how to sail in a sailboat that she had. It was just a small sailboat, a thirteen-foot sloop, but it was wonderful. When we were sailing, all of the pressures of school, teenage life, and farm work were far from my mind. I don't really know what kind of pressures this woman had because she never discussed them with me, but the moment that the wind made a whooshing sound and snapped the mainsail and jib with a thrust of air, the look on her face was one of serenity. We rarely talked about problems that either one of us were having; our time together was to be spent forgetting those troubles.

Her world took on a different perspective, though, after she went to see her doctor about an open sore on her breast that did not heal. Unfortunately, twenty-five years ago women were not as well versed on the warning signs of breast cancer. Signs like, "Go get a mammogram once a year for the rest of your life," were not seen on billboards on the highways as they are now. So though this was a well-educated woman with a master's degree in psychology, she did not realize that bloody drainage from the nipple, a sore that would not heel, and a palpable mass in her breast meant major trouble and the beginning of what would be a major health experience for her and those who loved her.

When given the verdict of breast cancer, she was dumbfounded and perplexed. My mother was very concerned for her and I had a personal fear of losing her. People didn't talk about breast cancer then. You could say that she had cancer, but it was taboo to say that it was breast cancer. Thank heavens things are different now, at least within most social circles.

Miss Bertha had a total radical mastectomy and remained her cheerful, upbeat self most of the time. After she was home about a month after her surgery, she asked me to look at her scar to make sure that it was healing okay because there was still a small spot that was weeping a tiny amount of drainage each day. I remember her saying to me that she felt comfortable with me seeing it because I was going to be a nurse and would know if there was anything wrong. What I really think she was seeking that day was acceptance of her appearance and not a *medical* opinion about her incision. I had never seen someone's scar after a mastectomy before and did my best to maintain flat affect and not show shock. But I was shocked.

Her cancer was advanced enough that the surgeon felt the need to remove the breast, muscle, lymph nodes in the arm and axillary area, and a few ribs, which meant that skin had to be grafted to her chest wall to close the wound. I could literally see her heart beating. It was quite scary to me. Despite my inner feelings and my youth, I mustered up the courage to say I thought it "looked very good and was healing as anticipated." She was so pleased to hear me say those words that she hugged me very close despite the fact that, I'm sure, her chest was very tender.

Having someone who loved her accept her was a very important thing at that time. She was not blessed with a loving husband to endure such a medical crisis and therefore had to rely on individuals other than her spouse for emotional and spiritual support. Crises such as these, I find, either bond a marriage closer together or drive it further apart. I suppose that, for her, her marriage was somewhat of an experience. But what is that old saying? "Love may be blind, but the neighbors ain't" fits for many marriages. And perhaps they *were* happy with one another . . . they just didn't seem to demonstrate it to the public eye.

Miss Bertha got a breast prosthesis a few months after her surgery and seemed to be back to her old self again. I remember one day being at her home and going to use the bathroom. She was waiting for me outside in her bathing suit, ready to walk to the beach at the foot of their property. Lying on the bathroom counter was an object that looked like a thick jellyfish. I picked it up and then discovered that it must have been her prosthesis! It certainly didn't look like a breast to me, nor did it feel like a breast, but I never to this day asked her any questions about it. I was convinced, though, that the inventor of the device lacked an understanding of what a breast prosthesis should look and feel like and thought that someday, if I had the opportunity to influence the designers of the future, I would give them my opinion of what I thought a prosthesis should be like.

Miss Bertha had a friend who had had bilateral mastectomies done for cancer. She visited her as often as time would allow even though she lived out of state. She was a neighbor to a relative in New York and was a very likable lady. I had the opportunity to meet her on several occasions and found her to be much like Miss Bertha—able to get on with her life despite the experiences life had dealt her. She and Miss Bertha acted different when they were with one another. Their behavior was hard to explain, but one could see the difference on their faces and hear it in their voices. They took great pleasure in telling funny stories about things that had happened to them individually in regards to their breast cancer. I'd like to share two of these twenty-year-old stories with you now.

The first one is about Miss Bertha's friend. She told us that after she had the second mastectomy, she realized that she could now be whatever bra size she wanted to be. She bought an inflatable bra and was very happy with it for a time. It was lightweight and allowed her to do her gymnastics routines that she enjoyed. One day she was flying out of town to visit a family member some distance away and as always had her inflatable bra on. Prior to her surgery, she was a very buxom woman, so she usually had her bra inflated to the max. This was apparently an unwise move in preparing for a plane flight.

There are lots of signs up in an airplane instructing you to do certain things and not to do certain things. You know—signs that tell you where the exits are, signs that tell you not to smoke. There is even a live demo or video movie of what to do in the event of a crash. But there are no signs that say, "If you are wearing an inflatable bra, we strongly recommend that you deflate it before takeoff or the pressure in the cabin will cause it to explode."

Yes, you guessed it. They were airborne about fifteen minutes; she was having a conversation with the man in the seat next to her when suddenly—*POW POW*—her bra exploded. Despite this shocking occurrence (or, I should say experience), she made believe that nothing had happened, slipped on her sweater that had been in her lap, and buttoned it up. When the opportunity presented itself, she scurried to the restroom and used tissues to fill what the atmospheric pressure had deflated.

She merely chalked it up to an experience in the life of a breast cancer survivor. Good for her!

The second story that I wanted to share is one that happened to Miss Bertha just a few months after her mastectomy. She was having a lot of trouble getting full range of motion back into her arm, so she decided to take up golf. She always found it a little silly to be walking up the walls with her fingers, which was the standard rehab exercises for mastectomy patients. She wanted to find a way that she could regain her range of motion and feel like her time spent doing it had not been wasted. Of course I know of some people who find hitting a little white ball around a field of green grass equally as productive as climbing up a wall with your fingers, but she was not one of those people. Anyway, she decided that she would need to have a golfing instructor to teach her the proper techniques in golf, so she signed up for lessons.

The instructor was totally unaware of why she had decided to take up golf and just assumed as anyone would that she was interested in this as a new sport. He was not very pleased with her progress, though, and was constantly telling her to "swing all the way through." One day, about four weeks into her private lessons, she *did* swing all the way through as he wanted and out fell her breast prosthesis onto the grass. (This predates when bras were available with pockets to put the prosthesis in.) She said that she looked at the object lying on the ground as if it had landed there from outer space. She couldn't bring herself to pick it up because she didn't want him to know that it was hers and worst of all to know *what* it was. He took the initiative and picked it up for her. As he handed it to her, he said, "Why didn't you tell me that you've had a mastectomy? I need to teach you different techniques to get your full swing." How marvelous that this man took the steps necessary to make her feel perfectly comfortable with herself and even more importantly with him. I never met him, nor do I know his name, but I instantly admired him after she told me this story.

I mentioned that both of these people acted differently when they were together and I want to explain more about that. It wasn't that they acted weird or anything, although Miss Bertha was known for doing funny things in strange places (like skipping down Fifth Avenue in New York City). It was that there was a special connection that the two of them seemed to make spiritually and emotionally when in each other's presence. I've seen this kind of special connection among babies who are twelve to eighteen months old and see one another in a stroller passing in the aisle of a department store. I have also seen it once when two children with Down's syndrome met by chance on a street corner and, having spotted one another, felt the need to hug one another though they did not know each other. They clearly recognized, despite their unfortunate intellectual disabilities, that they had something very special in common—something that no one but one of their own kind can share. As a breast cancer survivor now, myself, I now know what that special connection feels like that Miss Bertha and her friend shared. Truly it is special and only for club members. To be a club member, you must have or have had breast cancer. It is obviously an elite club and not one that you will find membership forms for in the back of a high-society magazine.

About ten years after Miss Bertha was originally diagnosed and treated for breast cancer, she had a recurrence in the form of bone cancer. It was at that time that she told me she had always wanted to have a child of her own but had not been blessed with the opportunity. She had been pregnant once but miscarried at five months. She felt as though I were the child whom she had never bore, and when we were in public, she admitted to me that, if someone asked if I was her daughter, she would tell them yes. She was glad to have me as her "borrowed" daughter and was now thankful that I wasn't her daughter by blood. She said that she would have felt very distressed if she had increased my risk of getting breast cancer. How strange that, even though we were not tied by blood, I would become a member of this elite club. Now I must deal with the guilt and fear that this defiant disease may have passed on to my child.

Both Miss Bertha and her friend have passed away now. Their survival as recoverers of breast cancer must not have been meant to be permanent, but they truly made the most of their lives and touched the hearts of many who knew them.

Chapter 2

My three years at Easton Memorial Hospital as a student nurse gave me ample time and opportunity to meet and provide nursing care to other club members who were diagnosed long before me. The first experience I can recall having with a mastectomy patient was during my nursing rotation in the recovery room. It was common practice in the late 1960s and early 1970s to go into surgery not even knowing if you were going to have just a biopsy or the whole ball of wax done to you all at once. Patients were asked to sign consent forms that in essence said that a breast biopsy was going to be done and if the frozen section pathology results showed it was cancer, then while the patient was still under anesthesia, the mastectomy would be performed as well. Of course, if the biopsy was negative then the patient would not have further surgery done that day as there would be none needed.

From the viewpoint of the people scheduling the operating room, gathering the necessary surgical supplies, and arranging for other things that would be needed to perform the second surgical procedure, it was all a matter of paperwork and stocking of shelves. But for the patient, it was fear of the unknown in the literal sense: going under the knife and not knowing until when you have awakened whether you had both breasts or not. This truly had to be like living a nightmare.

I recall the first patient that I took care of in the recovery room following a breast biopsy that was immediately followed by a total radical mastectomy. She awakened with a look of absolute terror on her face. As I checked her blood pressure, she grabbed my hand and asked in a frightened voice, "Tell me. Is it there? Is it gone? I don't want it to be gone. Please tell me that it isn't gone." My eyes connected with hers in a way that branded the image of her frightened face in my mind. My silence told her the answer that she didn't want to hear. Her sobbing could be heard like the cry of a trapped and injured animal. All I could think of to say was that I was sorry. I was sorry for her and, I guess, sorry for me—sorry that her worst fears had been realized and sorry for me that I was the one to be the bearer of bad news, even though I never really confirmed to her that she had had a mastectomy and that more awful treatment for her advanced breast cancer was to follow. She cried. I cried.

Of course, there were also those patients who awakened with that same horrified look but were given good news. "Yes, your breast is still there. Your doctor will be in shortly to talk with you." These women were so elated to have confirmed for them that "it" was still there that they felt no post-surgical pain upon hearing the good news. Their behavior was one of euphoric laughter and happiness, as if I had told them that while they were under anesthesia their lottery ticket had just won them ten million dollars.

That actually brings up an interesting point. What is the value of a breast, anyway? Some women pay a lot of money and suffer a lot of pain to have their breasts made bigger; others have had extensive and often risky surgery (such as a tram-flap procedure) to have a breast recreated from other parts of their own flesh to "replace" the one lost to cancer. And there are others who have had no surgery done to replace that which was stolen from them by this dreaded disease. Is this because a breast has no value? Or is it because the woman values it so much that a substitute or an imitation is considered to be worthless. I suppose this must be true because there are many women who have opted to have a lumpectomy rather than a mastectomy even if their doctor tells them that the risks of recurrence was greater by doing it this way. There are even some who have refused surgical intervention because the price of losing their breast is more than they can bear; these are women who often sacrifice their own life to avoid being, as they see it, dismembered.

I recall reading in *The Breast Book,* by Dr. Susan Love, that, for women in many cultures, breasts have had a deep, often mythological significance. Breasts to them are the external badge of womanhood. While the uterus is the center of reproduction, it is invisible; it does not identify us to the outside world as female. When we see an androgynous-looking person, we instinctively glance at the chest to determine the person's gender. Sexual attractiveness is also usually correlated to breast size—the larger the better, a concept represented in the media. A buxom chest has become a visible and outward symbol of femininity and sexuality. Yet you won't find women walking through grocery-store aisles stark naked from the waist up, showing off their femininity; this would not be socially acceptable (and thank heavens not, in my opinion).

This "let's see them—no you can't" attitude has added to society's confusion about how to deal with the topic of breast disease. Though the survivor club is growing, we still have a long way to go before people in general are comfortable talking with one another about cancers that affect particularly sensitive subject areas like breasts and testicles.

Perhaps the next generation, the one that my child is in, will deal with this issue differently. They are exposed to sexually explicit information now at a young age because of our need to prepare them for the pitfalls and risks of being sexually active (particularly AIDS). As a result, children know more about sex in elementary school than I did when I was first married at the age of twenty. Though I find that depressing and frightening, I do hope that these children will mature into young adults who are aware of the importance of good health, risk prevention, and openness with one another to discuss their fears of certain illnesses like breast cancer.

Five years ago, I discovered a lump in my right breast. I was thirty-four years old and very frightened when I found it one morning in the shower. I contacted my doctor and he scheduled me for a mammogram for the next day. I decided not to say anything to my coworkers partly because I didn't know them very well. I was about to be promoted into a new job and would be leaving the department anyway. I didn't feel comfortable telling the fellow wolves (all men) that I might have a serious problem with my breast. I went during lunchtime and, knowing the trip to the radiology building and back would probably take longer than an hour, I arranged to work late that evening.

I arrived in the mammography suite and could feel sweat running straight down between my cleavage. My nerves were shot just thinking of what they might tell me after they took the pictures. That was my first mistake. I expected to be *told* the answer immediately. If I had the pictures taken at the hospital where I worked, that probably would have happened, but I was in a strange place and answers were not forthcoming as I had hoped.

First the receptionist gave me a clipboard and asked me to fill out all of the forms on it. These included standard insurance papers, but there was also a special diagram of a woman's breast that needed to be completed. The instructions said to check "yes" or "no" to a long series of medical questions. Then the papers instructed me to draw on a diagram where I felt the lump. I checked "yes" to drainage from my nipple because since my child was born I had always retained milk. Even though I had not breast-fed her, I still had milk in my left breast and she was in third grade at this time. I used to joke with one of my friends that I could be a wet nurse. In any case, I answered "yes" to this question. There was no space to write down that the drainage was milk and there was no place to record that it was coming from the breast that felt fine. I then drew on the diagram where I felt the lump.

Next I was taken into the x-ray room and the mammogram was done. The first time a woman has a mammogram is probably the one she remembers the most vividly. When the technician picked up my left breast and placed it on the x-ray shelf, I felt as if she were scooping up a bag of marbles. Then the fun part came—the part where they try to see if it is *really* possible to take a large, round, dense mound of flesh and turn it into a one-quarter-inch-thick pancake. The answer to this question is yes, but it hurts like hell. The technician released the vice and did the same routine to the right breast. This was the side that I was worried about and it hurt even worse than the first one did in the smashing machine. Surely this radiology device was invented by a man who was still very angry with his mother because she refused to breast feed him. The technician then asked me to wait in the dressing room while the doctor looked at my pictures. This is what I had been waiting for; I wanted to be *with* the doctor when she looked at my films. I was told to wait, however.

When I got in the dressing room, the first thing I did was look at my breasts. I had the sudden irrational fear that when I picked up my hospital gown, I would see two humongous flat pancakes hanging from my chest. Relieved, I put my gown back down and waited. A few moments later the technician came and said, "You may get dressed now and go." Go? What did she mean, go? Certainly they wouldn't send me out the door without information about what the doctor saw. But they did. Despite my protests, despite my telling them that I was a nurse, they told me that my "doctor would be sent a report in the mail." Great. Now I'm also at the mercy of the United States Post Office.

I returned to work annoyed, but rationalized that if the doctor had seen anything that was worrisome, she would have said something or at least asked me more questions about my lump. I resolved myself to be satisfied to wait.

At 5:30 P.M., my phone rang. It was the doctor from the radiology building where I had just been a few hours earlier. Everyone from my immediate office area had gone for the day to begin the long holiday weekend, so I had some privacy to talk. She was calling because she said that she wanted more information about how long the lump had been there, whether I had been having any bloody drainage, if there was any dimpling of my breast, and whether I had any history of breast cancer in my family. I became very upset.

First of all, I had filled out those papers and all of these questions (except the *kind* of drainage) had been answered already. The doctor stated that she wanted to make sure of the information because of what she saw on the mammogram. Frightened, I asked her what she saw.

"I'm sorry, but I am not at liberty to discuss this with you. I will be having another radiologist look at the films on Monday and then we will be in touch with your doctor."

"What? You want me to wait to hear from my doctor? I can't wait! Tell me now!"

The doctor did not answer. She excused herself and hung up the phone. I started crying.

When I looked up a moment later a coworker from the department stood before me. He looked puzzled and concerned; he definitely wasn't ready for what was about to come out of my mouth. When he quietly inquired if I was all right, I responded by saying, "Oh, I don't know what I'm going to do. I think my boobs are going to fall off." This was obviously not the response he had anticipated. It was very unlike me to use such an expression. He also had no idea why I thought this strange phenomenon would happen to me. I explained to him how I had spent my lunch hour and he shared my concerns and anxieties of this unknown diagnosis. He helped me by trying to assist me in reaching my doctor, but the news only got worse. My doctor was on vacation until the following Wednesday; he had just left the office. His secretary said, "Oh, gee, you just missed him. You nearly missed me, too, because I was just locking up to leave." I felt completely defeated.

That was an awful weekend for me. It had been planned to be a very special one but those plans were ruined now. It was the following day that I was to graduate from Johns Hopkins University where I had finally completed my master's degree in administrative science. It was to be a happy time, a time of celebration. My folks were coming over for the ceremony. My husband Al and I decided that there was no reason to worry them with this health problem until we had it confirmed that it was a problem, so our concerns were kept a secret. It was a long weekend, an unpleasant and sleepless one.

On Wednesday of the following week I was successful in reaching my doctor and explained to him the alarming call that I had received from the radiology doctor just hours after having left her side. He promptly called her and then called me back. "Lillie, there is nothing to worry about. It's a blocked milk duct; hot compresses and antibiotics will fix you right up." A blocked milk duct? Then why did this female radiologist scare me to death? Well, come to find out, she was a resident in training and quite new at reading mammograms, which explained why she was having another doctor review them before a report was to be sent to my own doctor. All of that worrying was for nothing; my graduation weekend had been ruined because of it. Now that I look back on it, I feel that it was just a dress rehearsal for the real thing that would come five years later.

Chapter 3

My experience in 1988 with thinking that I had breast cancer caused me to reflect back to when I had cared for patients who went through the same awful experience—the awful waiting, not knowing, and always fearing the worst. My husband was also scared in 1988—scared for me. Scared for himself that he might lose me. We spent some time over that very long weekend talking about all of the what-ifs.

Question: *What if it is cancer and I have to have a mastectomy? Will you still love me?*
Answer: *Of course.*

Question: *What if I have to have chemotherapy and lose what is left of my hair. What will you think when you look at me?*
Answer: *I will see you as I do now—my wife whom I love very much . . .*

But God had been kind to me that time, sparing me the experience of having to prove these hypotheses. As I said before, it was just a dress rehearsal for a real experience. It gave me the chance to talk about it with the man whom I love so very much to see what his reactions would be.

Though we exchanged only verbal remarks, they meant a lot to me.

As I mentioned earlier, we had chosen not to tell my family, or for that matter anyone, until we knew the verdict. Why worry people we loved? They had enough of their own worries without me adding to them. So we told everyone that we had a scare but the scare was over. My folks were not pleased that they were not included from the start, however, and I promised them that if ever I had a scare again I would let them know about it early on so they could lose as much sleep as the rest of us did.

Never give up the opportunity to worry your parents. They expect it and will be angry with you if you don't. Somewhere there is an unwritten law that says parents must assume full responsibility for their offspring's well-being until parent or child dies. The assumption is that the parents will die first, not because they are old and decrepit, but because they worry themselves into an early grave. I share in the belief in this unwritten law because I have a daughter of my own and I can tell that I am going to worry about her and the various turns her life takes until I am pushing up daisies myself.

After about a month or so, I was able to stop thinking about my near experience with breast cancer and stop focusing on my breasts and their health status. The lump went away just as my doctor said it would and my life was back to its usual level of chaos. My respect for women who had had the real experience raised. I started using more Ivory soap in the house too, purely as a reminder that their slogan that year was a good take-home message. Their TV commercials were done by a young woman who grew up in the country and wore very little makeup. The woman stood there looking lovely and physically fit while her TV husband talked about how beautiful his wife's skin was. They closed the commercial with the slogan, "When you've got your health, you've got just about everything." Though I didn't think washing my breasts each day in the shower with Ivory soap would be some new form of preventive medicine for breast cancer, I did think it would remind me of the value of good health. We take for granted that which we have until we lose it. This experience also inspired me to have a cross-stitched piece of work that I had done in high school to be dug out my storage chest and professionally framed. It has a picture of a well on it and it says, "When the well is dry, we know the worth of water." I valued the appendages that hung from my chest all the more after that year.

Life was basically back to normal. During the same month that I had my mammography scare I was promoted to the position of director of quality assessment, utilization, and risk management at the Johns Hopkins Hospital where I had been working for five years. It was a very demanding job and required long hours and a lot of hard work. I still have that job and I take the responsibilities of this position very seriously. I am a highly driven person, and I love my work. The pace and demands of my job made it easy to forget about my scary experience the month before. Time passed quickly, and before I knew it, it was 1992.

In April of 1992, I began to have pain in my right breast. It was the same side that I had had the blocked milk duct in before, so I wasn't very worried about it. I decided to use the warm compress treatment I had used before, but this time it didn't work. So after three weeks of no relief, I decided to call the doctor and he ordered a mammogram.

The mammogram was done at the hospital where I worked. Because of my position there I personally know the majority of the physicians there. Also because of my position I am fortunate to get prompt service and medical care usually at a moment's notice. (I personally feel, though, that the care at Hopkins is the best in the country whether you have access to special contact people there or not.)

The mammogram was done by a mammography technician named Robin who was very compassionate and caring. She was really in the right line of business; I felt very much at ease with her. I told her I had concluded, after having had this second mammogram done, that if ever the United States was to go to war again, I knew the perfect weapon. The military should be provided portable mammogram machines. Forget about M-16 rifles. Just let them carry one of these metal vices. When a soldier catches an enemy, he can put a three-piece set on him and crunch vital organs as a technician would a woman's breast. Whatever military secrets the enemy might know would soon be revealed. (My husband had later said that they could call it a gonadogram weapon.)

She completed the procedure and asked me to wait in the booth for the films to be checked. I asked whether a particular radiologist whom I know well would be available to read the films *with* me. I thought that there was no reason for me to wait for the verdict again. I'd prefer to discuss the results of these films right away. Anyway, I was sure that the problem was minor, something similar to what I had the last time in 1988. Luck was with me; the radiologist came into the room a few moments later.

Unfortunately, he said there was a cyst in the right breast which was probably what was causing me pain. He paused a moment and said there was also something that appeared on the films taken of my left breast. There were calcified areas he wanted to take a closer look at. Calcified areas? Well, I decided not to worry until he gave me more information after additional films of my breast were taken.

Robin reappeared and took a few more pictures of the left side. About half an hour went by before the radiologist reappeared. He told me that there was definitely something there, but that enlargments of the films showed the calcifications to be spherical, which is usually a good sign. However, their pattern was in the shape of a horseshoe and they were in the process of closing into a circle; because of this, he felt it wise to have me be seen by a breast surgeon for an opinion about the area. I felt reassured, though, because he said that the possibility of this being cancer was extremely slim. Thank heavens, I thought. Also the radiologist was a comforting, gentle man who stands tall and stoic and has a marvelous calming effect on nervous patients like myself. So I left the radiology department feeling very little concern.

Over that weekend, my gynecologist called me at home and said he was at the hospital and had received a copy of my mammogram. He shared the radiologist's opinion and recommended that I go see a breast surgeon. He decided that I could choose my surgeon because of the business I was in.

I asked one of my employees whom she felt was a good breast surgeon. The surgeon she mentioned was an excellent choice based on the information available to me. He had a reputation for being an excellent surgeon among the hospital staff. The length of stay for his breast cancer patients was also shorter than most, which was a plus in my book. (Being responsible for utilization management at the hospital causes me to look at patient care clinically and financially. Shorter lengths of stay are more medically optimal now and are usually better for the patient and her pocketbook.) He was also considered to be an excellent surgeon by the operating nurses and floor nurses; he was known to be compassionate, caring, and very thorough. I knew that I would be in good hands. His name was Charlie Yeo.

I was able to get an appointment with Dr. Yeo the same week. He was as impressive in person as his paper credentials and feedback from other health care professionals had said he would be. After being with him only a few moments, I thought about how much he reminded me of my brother—a straightforward, charismatic precisionist.

He examined my breasts then showed me my mammography films and pointed out where the cyst was on the right breast and where the calcified area was in the left breast. He felt, as the radiologist had, that this was probably nothing to worry about, but that it would be wise to do an open biopsy of the calcified area. At the same time he would do a needle aspiration of the cyst in the right breast. I still felt very calm about the whole thing and left the exam room feeling that this procedure would be no big deal. Whatever the calcified area was, it had to be removed so that it wouldn't create trouble for me later in life, and the drainage of the cyst would be a piece of cake.

I contacted Dr. Yeo's secretary; she got me booked for the minor surgery to be done in the outpatient center on the second of June. When I got home that evening I told my husband the plans and he too felt there was nothing to worry about. I contacted my mother that evening and told her what was happening so she could spend three full weeks getting worried about it. And she did. So did my dad.

On June 2, 1992, I arrived at the outpatient center for the procedure to be done. The medical director of ambulatory care was talking with a patient in the booth next to me. He spotted me right away. He was surprised to see me and checked on me several times to make sure things were going as planned that day.

The full name of the procedure was called a "breast biopsy with needle localization" and I would sum it up in one word: yuck. The beginning of the procedure involved having my left breast placed back into the mammography machine and once again smashed down until it resembled a wad of dough. Then the fun part came.

A radiologist came in and inserted a needle into my breast that was to serve as a guide for the surgeon to find the calcified lesion. She used the x-ray as her guide to find the spot in question and inserted the needle. While doing the procedure she said something that would soon result in a few moments of chaos in the room. She explained that it was hard to push the needle in while my breast was compressed in the mammogram machine; the density of the tissue combined with the compression made it difficult. I didn't know what to say or do, maybe because I was too scared.

Picture it. My breast is being held captive by a ton of metal that has a vice on it and I have a needle hanging out of my breast. I kept thinking about it, and thinking about it more, which was a mistake. I glanced down and watched her as she tried to get the needle farther into the breast. That did it. Looking. Watching the needle go in. And, oh no . . . I started seeing spots before my eyes. The wall in front of me that had been a lovely shade of orchid now was snow white. Then everything went white. I said, "I'm in trouble. I think I'm going to faint." That's what caused the chaos.

A blood pressure cuff was quickly obtained and people hastened around to get me in a chair. Ironically enough I don't think that I would have actually fallen. How could I? My breast was still in the vice. I couldn't have landed on the floor if I had tried. Smelling salts were stuck under my nose and I was placed in a cardiac lounge chair and my feet were propped up. After a few minutes the wall returned to its original shade of orchid and my face was flushed from embarrassment.

Even though people tell you that an embarrassing event could have happened to anybody, it didn't happen to just anybody. It happened to me. I'm a nurse and have seen everything from gunshot wounds to the head to open trauma of the chest, and even accidental limb amputations. All of that never bothered me. But, of course, none of those patients were me. It's different if it is you, or someone you love a great deal, like your own child. Then the event is more unpredictable because you don't know how you are going to react.

She finished this part of the procedure by injecting blue dye in through the needle. The dye marked the area for the surgeon to excise. Soon I was taken into an area where I would wait to be carted into the surgical suite. My husband, Al, was able to be with me in this waiting area. That was reassuring. The needle was still hanging out of my breast; a cup was placed over it and taped in place. I disliked having the procedure done, but knew it was one of the most precise ways to pinpoint an abnormal area for the surgeon to excise. The wait was brief and shortly thereafter I was escorted into the surgery room.

Once on the table, I knew the show was soon to begin. Dr. Yeo came in already scrubbed and ready to go. He first drained the cyst in the right breast, which only took a few seconds, then concentrated his efforts on the real job at hand. I was very nervous and couldn't stop talking. The nurses in the room with me were very accommodating and allowed me to ramble on about the weather, vacation plans, and other such nonsense. The surgeon injected me with local anesthetic numerous times. Unfortunately, my experience in the dentist's office has always been that I require a lot of that stuff before I'm genuinely numb. So was the case on this day. Periodically I would wince or say ouch and he would give me another shot in the breast area. Dr. Yeo said that he was surprised to find that I had severe cystic disease and that he had drained six cysts before he got to the location of the blue dyed area. The tissue mass that was removed was gray. Some good tissue was taken out as well for pathology to inspect. The procedure took about forty-five minutes, but it felt like two hours. Finally I was stitched closed and the dressing was applied.

We were allowed to leave the hospital an hour later. Dr. Yoe told me as we left that he would be out of town for a few days and when he returned he would call me with the results. He didn't want me to worry, though, and I didn't.

Al and I got home at about 2:30 that day. I felt pretty good. My mother had come over earlier in the day because Laura, our daughter, had stayed home from school with a tummy ache. I suspected that it was due to worrying about her mother, and it was. Laura doesn't like to hear that someone has to have a shot, much less an operation.

My mother was glad to see me. She looked as I imagined she would. Worried. Caring. Loving. Patient. She also had an expression on her face that confirmed for me that she had a whopper of a migraine headache. And why shouldn't she? Remember, I gave her three whole weeks to worry about that day's events. She stayed until about six P.M. then headed home to the farm, a two-hour drive away.

I stayed home from work the next two days, which was not what I had originally planned. The local anesthetic wore off at around seven P.M. and I felt like someone had struck me in the chest with a baseball bat. I was also alarmed to see my incision. It wasn't what I had expected. But then again, the amount of diseased breast tissue that the surgeon had to remove was more than he had expected he would.

The incision was about three and one half inches long and it indented into my breast. When I raised my hand up over my head, it indented in even farther and I started to cry. Al comforted me and told me that I looked fine. That was the first time I realized that I was body-image conscious about my breasts.

My secretary, Diane, came from work the next day to bring me some papers I wanted to work on at home over the weekend. Marge, one of my other staff, had been there at seven A.M. to drop off some other work material I had finished by the time that Diane had arrived. Diane is a special person to me. She's not just a great secretary, she is also a very dear friend. Having her visit for a while and exchanging with her the completed work that I had done that morning helped me feel productive. Her visit also reinforced in my mind how much she cared about and loved me.

Diane went to work that Saturday so I decided not to wait until Dr. Yeo was back in town. I had access to my medical record in the pathology database at work so I asked Diane to check the results of my biopsy. Why wait to get good news? I was sure that the mass would be benign. Remember, it was calcified *circles,* not irregular in size. I had just had preventive surgical care done, I thought. Certainly this was not the beginning of an experience, but the end of one. The path report wasn't ready, though, so I was unable to get a preview of this good news after all.

On Monday I went to work. My staff were all supportive and empathetic. They too were anxious for me to get the good news so that their anxiety could be relieved. Still, however, the report wasn't ready.

On Tuesday afternoon I checked the database again. This time it said that the specimen had been sent to another pathologist for verification. Come on, people. Why is it taking so long to get this good news on my computer screen? Tuesday evening came and many of my staff had been in and out of my office asking if I had the report results yet. Still the answer was no.

Right before I got ready to leave, Diane, who was there late with me, said, "The report is back. I checked it an hour ago. I wanted you to have privacy when you read it. I don't understand what it said."

I logged on and pulled it up onto the screen. It contained the usual medical terminology. It contained words like "specimen," "tissue," and "cells." Then I read words that I was not prepared to read on a report with my name on it: "intraductal carcinoma." I read it over and over and still the same words appeared. The expression "out of the margins" also haunted me as I read more. I quickly logged off and asked Diane to go into the database with her password, thinking that it would tell her something different—not rational thinking on my part, but who thinks rationally when in shock? I had hoped that when she pulled my report up on the screen, it would say, "Ha! Ha! Fooled you! That will teach you to look at your own report rather than wait for your doctor to call you on Wednesday." But that wasn't what it said. The words all looked the same as before. It was cancer.

Diane was very upset but kept her cool. She said that the doctor had taken the mass out, so there was nothing to worry about. I told her I wasn't so sure because it said that it was "out of the margins," which meant that there were still cancer cells in the breast. She hurriedly went to our other office down the hall and brought me back our medical journals and reference books. While she did that, I copied the report down on paper and stared at the words before me. My head was swimming with images of awful things yet to come. Could this be a secondary metastasis from another primary site? Was it in both breasts? Was it in my lymph nodes? Was I going to die? What could I do to make this awful experience go away? I logged off the computer and stared at the dark, blank screen as if I were looking at the grim reaper.

The textbooks were somewhat helpful because they refreshed my memory from my clinical nursing days; for the majority of patients diagnosed with breast cancer, intraductal carcinoma was *not* a death sentence. I wrote down information from these books too and packed up my briefcase. Diane kissed me good-bye. She looked very worried—worried for her friend and trying to figure out how she could make all of this awfulness go away.

I walked down the corridors toward the parking-lot exit. One of the hallways that I passed and have walked by probably ten thousand times was the corridor that led to the oncology center. I caught myself walking faster than usual to avoid thinking about having to enter those doors as a patient in the near future, perhaps even fearing that the doors would spontaneously open as I walked by and a great vacuum would suck me in. Finally I made it to the car. Once I was alone, I began to cry.

I turned on the radio very loud and pushed in a cassette tape of Natalie Cole's "Unforgettable." Music has always been a great soother for me and singing with music I have always found to be very therapeutic. I sang and cried and sang some more. I knew that when I got home my husband would not be there because of work. He had driven a limousine to New York City to drop off some people who had rented it for the day. He was not expected back until around nine P.M. I knew Laura would be there but I didn't want to upset her—I didn't want her to know that anything was wrong. I pulled myself together and parked the car in the driveway.

Laura could tell I had been crying. She wanted to know what was wrong. I told her I had had a bad day at work and not to worry about it. She wanted to eat dinner. We had planned to go out for a "girl's dinner" since her daddy wasn't going to be home in time to eat with us. I told her I couldn't go out, though. I didn't feel well and wanted to stay home, hoping that Al would get home sooner than planned. Her inquisitive mind persisted; she kept asking me if I was all right. I guess I wasn't very convincing that the problems on my face were solely work related. My brain was working on overdrive trying to figure out how to tell my husband, how to tell my parents, and how and when to tell my child. My head ached and I couldn't erase the vision of the computer screen with those words typed out so plain and cold: carcinoma of the breast.

Chapter 4

Laura got herself ready for bed at a quarter past eight. She went to sleep unknowing of the crisis at hand. I felt very relieved when she went to bed because at least I had succeeded in sparing her a restless and nightmarish night. It gave me some comfort to know that she could rest unburdened by concerns about her mother's health.

The phone rang shortly thereafter and I hoped desperately that it was Al calling me from the limo car phone. I picked up the receiver and said hello. It was my mother.

"Do you know anything yet?" she asked. I was frozen in place and unable to speak. My silence gave her the answer just as my silence had given the verdict to that first mastectomy patient I had taken care of so very many years ago. I told her that Al wasn't home yet and I'd rather call her back after he got home. I spoke softly so I wouldn't awaken Laura. Mom didn't want the conversation to end there, though. She wanted answers and asked me again about the path report.

"Is it bad?" I paused a few seconds, answered yes, and started to cry. I grabbed the portable phone and walked outside so Laura would not be disturbed.

My mother was now in shock. I felt thankful that I didn't have to see her face at that moment. I knew how distressed she must have felt and direct eye contact then would have been more than my heart could have handled. I told her I would call her back in twenty minutes and I hung up the phone. Time was motionless. I wanted the clock to hasten forward so that my husband would be home with me. At the same time, I wanted the clock to go slowly so that I would have time to pull myself together and figure out how I was going to tell him I had cancer. I also wanted to figure out what to tell my mother when I called her back that would make her feel better. I searched for something I could say that would let her know that I would get through this . . . that we'd all get through this. The problem, though, was that I wasn't sure that I *would* get through this, that I would survive this dreadful and potentially deadly experience. All I knew was that I had breast cancer. I didn't know what stage it was in. I didn't know exactly what the treatment would be. I assumed that I would need a mastectomy, but I wasn't absolutely sure of anything. I was able to collect myself; I called my mother back about five or ten minutes later.

Her voice sounded strained. I worried about how she was going to deal with my telling her that I knew very little but what I knew was bad. Having to tell her that I had read my report and it indicated breast cancer was like pouring acid into her ears right through the phone. She was very upset that I that I'd have to wait until I went to work in the morning and spoke to Dr. Yeo to get any definitive answers. She told me that she loved me and I told her the same. It sounded different somehow—more tangible than I ever remembered hearing it sound before, more intense. I told her that when Al got home I'd have him call her again after I talked with him. She said okay and the conversation ended.

Al called on the car phone only a few minutes later. I was very steady on the phone with him and tried not to project over the telephone lines that I was in major trouble. I didn't want him to get the news the way my mother had because he was driving. I would be even more distressed if I would have said or done anything that jeopardized his safety behind the wheel. Our conversation was brief. He told me that he would be home in about twenty minutes and began telling me about the day he had. I really didn't hear much of what he said. I just clung to the words, "I'll be home in twenty minutes," and once again I wanted time to race by swiftly so he could be home with me.

At a quarter to ten he walked through our kitchen door. He was very tired. He said he was hungry and began to go to the fridge. I stopped him and asked him to go downstairs to the basement with me. He looked very perplexed by such an odd request and asked me why, but I just repeated my request to come downstairs. He followed me down the steps. At the bottom of the staircase I stood in front of him and said, "I saw my path report. I have breast cancer." There. I'd done it. He knew. I was relieved to have the words out of my mouth.

Al looked at me in shock and said, "Well that doesn't mean that it's malignant, does it?" I nodded yes. He grabbed me and squeezed me very tight. That moment will live on in my memory for the rest of my life. I could feel his strength around me and knew that if it was possible to beat this, I could do it with his love. What he couldn't do for me was make it all go away.

It was like a bad dream—a dream that I wanted to wake up from but couldn't. To complicate matters, Al had to return the limousine that night because the company needed it for a morning run. I didn't want him to go. He didn't want to leave either. First I thought I could go with him, then I remembered that Laura was in bed, so I stayed behind. He promised to hurry back. When he left I felt a sense of panic. He said he'd be back within the hour. He told me that he loved me three times.

What was I to do with myself until he returned? Not just sit in a chair and wait. I had done enough of that already and it made me feel worse. I decided to empty the dishwasher. Upon completing that task, I scrubbed out the shower in the master bathroom. "Well, if I'm going to die from cancer anytime soon," I thought, "I might as well have a clean house." I pictured people coming to my funeral and saying, "She sure went down fast. Gee, from diagnosis to death in only a week. But you know, her kitchen and bathroom looked and smelled really clean." I remember glancing at the bar of Ivory soap and decided to replace it with Coast soap, my previous favorite. The Ivory went into the trash.

Al returned within the hour, just as he had promised. He walked through the door at 11:20 P.M. He told me that he didn't even remember driving down the beltway to Sandy's house where he returned the limousine. Clearly his brain must have been on auto pilot to have brought him safely there and back to me. But the important thing was that he was back home, and all that I desired at that moment was his arms around me. As he and I stood in the kitchen, holding each other tightly, I thought, "Protect me; make this awful thing go away." But I knew this was not possible for him to do for me. I also knew that he too was frightened but desperately was trying not to show it. We both knew that this time this experience was not a dress rehearsal as it had been four years earlier. This time it was the real thing.

He called my folks as I had promised my mother he would. I don't know what they said to him, but he was remarkably steady on the phone with them. Amazingly steady. Confident. Confident that we would get through this experience. Confident that I would do well. Just hearing him tell them these words made me feel better. "Of course he's right. Of course I will. Please, God, make him dead right about this, because if he's dead wrong, then I'm dead," I thought.

We went to bed at half past midnight. Not many words were spoken in our house after he hung up the phone with my parents. We got undressed, turned off the lights, and held each other like two shipwrecked survivors who were riding out a furious storm. The date was June 9, 1992, the day I found out that I had just been involuntarily drafted into the club.

I rose early and went in to work the next morning. My first mission was to call Dr. Yeo's office and get more information about my future, my life. His secretary answered the phone and told me that he was returning that day from having been out of town and would probably be in late. My heart sank. I explained to her that I had pulled up my path report on the computer and I needed to discuss the results with him right away. She said that their office had not received that report yet. I told her it was imperative that I talk with him because I knew that I had cancer. She told me that she would put my file on the very top of his pile of work to review and would print off a copy of the path results for him to see. I thanked her and hung up. I must have stared at that phone for two or three minutes before I could get on with my day. I relayed to Diane, my secretary, what the status of my phone call was and she agreed to find me wherever I might be when he called me back.

I tried to clear my head. I had work to be done and needed to get on with my day. Sitting by a phone to wait for it to ring would have turned me into a crazy person.

I went on with my meetings. My first meeting was with one of my bosses, Dr. Timothy Townsend. I had my usual list of issues to discuss and make decisions about and our meeting went on without him having a clue that anything was wrong in my life. As our meeting ended and I left his office, Carole, his secretary and a longtime friend, greeted me and handed me a long-stemmed rose with a card that said, "Thinking of you and hoping for the best." Carole was aware that I had a biopsy but was unaware that I already knew the verdict. At least she was unaware until I made eye contact with her.

I stood before her silently and tears began to flow down my face. I couldn't stop them. My silence continued. No words were needed. She promptly rushed over to hug me. With that, Tim came out of his office. He asked whether I knew the results of my biopsy. I nodded yes but could not bring myself to speak. After a moment of total silence, I said, "The biopsy was positive. I have breast cancer." Tim asked what Dr. Yeo had told me would be the next step. Then I floored him by telling him that Dr. Yeo didn't know the results yet and that I looked them up on the computer myself. Both Carole and Tim were very supportive. Carole felt bad that she caused me to cry. I had arrived at their office looking fine and upon receiving a rose turned into a basket case. Heaven only knows what I would have done if she had handed me a lily. Tim walked me back to my office. He has a warm, genuinely caring manner and has a wonderful way with patients. He told me to call him as soon as I heard from Dr. Yeo. He hugged me at my office door and departed.

Now that I was back in my office, several of my staff were anxious to know if I had my path results yet. As people came in and asked me my path results, I mustered up the strength to tell them that it was positive. Everyone was in shock. Everyone wanted to know the next step and hoped that no further treatment was needed. "He took out the lesion, so that should be all." That was the response from the majority. I knew in my heart that more treatment was to come. I could feel it within me. The report had said it was "outside the margins." This meant that there were still cancer cells left in the breast.

The day dragged along despite a fairly full schedule. At three P.M. Tim came by to check on me.

"Any news?"

"No, I still haven't heard from the surgeon's office yet."

I decided to call his office again and hoped that I wouldn't be misrepresented as a pest. I thought if I was labeled as a pest maybe that would make the doctor mad and he'd want to take my arm off along with my breast. Isn't it just awful the crazy things that we think of when our brain is one place and our body is in another?

Tracy, his secretary, answered the phone as she had before. "I hate to bother you or Dr. Yeo, but do you know when he will be able to talk with me?" The response was not what I had expected. "Gee, Mrs. Shockney, I'm really sorry. He was only briefly here and is gone right now. He'll be in touch with you in the morning." The morning? I didn't think that I would mentally make it another eighteen hours. She said, "He wants to discuss the path report with the pathologists and with another breast surgeon."

I felt like Dorothy in the *Wizard of Oz*. Remember when she was abducted by flying monkeys, had her dog taken away from her by the evil witch, was locked in a room with only minutes to live and, despite a myriad of obstacles, managed to defeat the wicked witch of the west? The deal that she had made with the Great Oz was that if she brought him the witch's broom, he would get her home to Kansas. Well, she brought him the broom and what did he say? He told her, "Come back tomorrow." Tomorrow was forever to me. Can you imagine telling a woman in hard labor to just keep panting until tomorrow? She'd punch your lights out. But I had no one to punch. I was too wasted to fight with anybody.

I tried to fantasize that maybe he could talk the pathologists into changing their minds and rewriting the path report. He could say, "Hey fellows, this lady is really nice. How about lightening up a little and rewording that report to say, 'Great-looking breast tissue. Looks like it belongs to the body of a twenty-five-year-old. No abnormalities found.'"

The evening dragged on. Al and I talked a lot and I told him I was ninety-nine percent sure that my surgeon would be recommending a mastectomy. I was really scared of how he would react to such a surgical procedure. I kept saying to him, "You don't know what this kind of scar will look like. The breast will be totally gone. Do you understand me? Gone. I will look awful. You might not want to look at me anymore."

He remained as steadfast that night as he had before and for that matter as he had four years before when we went through the awful dress rehearsal. "I want you well. I don't care what kind of surgery that you need. I love you. We'll get through this. I love you." Then he'd hold me again and I'd cry. We both felt like we were still in shock. I don't think that either one of us could believe that any of this was happening to me, to us. I'm not sure what my parents were going through at this point, still not knowing what the future held for their child.

This next day was June 11th. I had a meeting before work with a financial consultant to review my benefits and annuity arrangements that I had through the hospital. I had met this gentlemen once before at a seminar the hospital held for employees. His name was Bud Leeb. Bud is a very personable man. He came in intending to review my financial profile so I could do as I had planned to have him help me do: plan for my future, plan for my eventual retirement in twenty years. My retirement? Good heavens. It was not a very good day for me to be looking at that kind of information. I didn't even know if I would live to *see* retirement. I didn't feel like talking about finances. What I needed was a lawyer to update my will, I thought.

Bud was very cheerful and pleasant. I didn't want to ask him to leave and reschedule me. After all, he had traveled here from his office many miles away and I didn't want to impose on him again. So we proceeded with the meeting as planned. As he talked with me he was looking around my office and noticed a lot of cards and flowers. A lot of my staff had given me flowers and cards to lift my spirits. He said, "Gee, is it your birthday?" I told him that it wasn't. "Is it your anniversary or something?" I again answered no. "Well, it must be a special occasion because you sure have lots of beautiful flowers and cards." I disintegrated into tears. He was very alarmed and apologized for upsetting me and asked what was wrong.

I told him I had just found out that I had breast cancer and was waiting to hear from my doctor anytime now. He told me that his wife had been diagnosed with cancer many years ago and the doctor had given her a poor prognosis. She had a strong will to live and remained optimistic throughout her treatments and multiple abdominal surgeries. (She also obviously had a wonderful support system—her husband.) He told me that he had no business troubling me today with numbers; I was to concentrate on my health and be optimistic. He gave me a hug and left my office quite swiftly.

To think that he felt that he was troubling me...For goodness sake, I was the one who had made the appointment with him. About fifteen minutes later, my secretary came to my door with a basket of daisies and a card. They were from Bud. Bud from that day forward became a new friend and a member of my support system for the future.

At a quarter past eleven Diane came to my door and nervously said that it was Dr. Yeo on the phone. She closed my door.

This was the call that I had been waiting for. The little light blinking on my phone was the answer to my concerns about my life, my longevity, and my body. I picked up the phone and quickly grabbed a pen and paper.

"Mrs. Shockney, I hope that you're sitting down because I'm afraid I have bad news." Bad news? Didn't he know that I already knew that I had breast cancer? Unfortunately not. The message he received was lost in translation. He only knew I wanted to talk with him as a soon as possible about my biopsy results. He didn't know that I already knew what the path report said.

He was stunned that I had been aware for two days and realized now why I had placed two calls to his office. He explained to me that when he returned from his trip and reviewed the path report he wanted to talk directly with the pathologist about the findings. He met with Dr. Baker, a known expert at the hospital in the field of breast cancer, for a second opinion about the best treatment options for me. He recommended that I have a mastectomy. The second option was a lumpectomy with radiation. The third option was to do nothing at all. (This may not seem like an option, but it is a choice that a patient has the right to choose.) He suggested that I go home and discuss it with my husband. I interrupted him.

"What do you feel will give me the best chance of long-term survival? What would you tell me if I were your wife, your sister?"

"A mastectomy will give you the best long-term outcomes."

"When do you want me to go in for the surgery?"

He paused. "Don't you want to discuss this with your husband?" I explained that I already had and reminded him that I'd had two and a half days to think about this and was not surprised with his surgical recommendation.

I wrote down every word he said. *Every word*. I was proud of myself with how steady I was on the phone with him. Again I had the advantage of no required eye contact. I only choked up once and that's when we were discussing the date for surgery. He told me I was a strong woman and he was sorry I had to deal with this knowledge of knowing I had cancer and not knowing what the next step would be. I told him I regretted looking up the information on the computer, but having access to the database had been too tempting. And anyway, I felt sure it would be benign as was the prediction of physicians. He was very encouraging. I felt somewhat relieved to hear him recite statistics that sounded favorable to me from a longevity perspective.

When we discussed a surgery date, I explained that my husband and I had planned a vacation the first week of July. I wondered if I should cancel it. "Definitely not. By all means, get away for a few days. That way you'll be all rested up for surgery when you return." We agreed on July 14th. He originally suggested July 13th but I requested the following day. (July 13th was the day I married my first husband. My ex-husband. I had enough bad memories of that day and felt no need to add to them.) He gave me the number of a clinical nurse specialist to talk with me about the surgery and I recorded her name and number. Our conversation ended at this point.

Dr. Yeo was professional, charming, and, as always, thorough in providing me all the information I requested of him. I elected to tell him before he hung up that I was impressed with his thoroughness and the time he afforded me. It was physicians like him that made me proud to be the director of quality assessment and utilization management at the hospital.

Upon hanging up, Diane obviously saw the light go out on the phone and opened the door to my office. When I saw her come in, I started crying. She put her arms around me. She asked what he had said to me. "I'm scheduled for a mastectomy on July 14th." She cried even harder then. I think she cried harder and longer than I did. Though I felt upset I also felt relieved—relieved to know there was something that could rid me of this dreadful disease. I felt optimistic that the outcome would not be a lovely bronze box covered with flowers and confident that I was in the very best medical hands I could possibly be in.

I called Al and told him what Dr. Yeo had said to me. He was very positive. "Ninety-five to ninety-nine percent survival rate at ten years. Well, that sounds good to me. We're going to be okay, baby. I love you. It probably hasn't spread yet. That's a blessing. Even more to be relieved about. We'll get through this. We will. It will be okay. Do you want me to come and get you? Maybe you should be home. I just want to come and scoop you up and take you home with me and take care of you." I thought how God had surely blessed me with a good husband. He was truly a rock, and I needed him to be. I told him I was going to continue my work schedule and to not worry. I'd call him before I left at the end of the day.

Diane and I went to lunch. We only had about twenty-five minutes before my next meeting. It didn't matter because neither one of us had much of an appetite by then. My left breast ached as I walked down the hall—purely psychosomatic pain. It hadn't ached all day until then.

My one o'clock meeting was with a group of my staff. These were employees whom I had spent a lot of time with and felt especially close to. They had no idea yet that I had heard from the doctor. Only a few of them even knew at this point that my biopsy results were back. I didn't want to use this forum as the place to discuss my upcoming surgery. It was not an agenda item I had planned to discuss in an open meeting. I wanted to do that in private. I went into the restroom and tried to collect myself. "You can do this," I said to myself. "Just push this personal problem out of your mind and get on with business. This is not the place to blurt out that you're getting your breast removed." I took in deep breaths, composed myself, left the restroom, and entered the conference room door.

Everyone was there. I took my seat and began covering my preplanned agenda. As I covered each agenda item on my list and discussed each topic, I caught my mind wandering, though only for a few seconds at a time. I thought about how the people who were sitting before me had no idea what I had just been told. They had no idea that I had breast cancer and would be having my breast off the next month.

I felt a personal sense of pride that I was able to go on with business as usual. I was glad I was able to pull it off and felt hopeful I would be able to conduct my work without this personal crisis affecting my productivity. That was important to me.

When I returned to my office I wrote out notes to several members of my staff, whom I felt especially close to. I wrote that I had gotten the news from Dr. Yeo and that I was scheduled for a mastectomy. It was hard to write it on the paper. I looked at what I had written and couldn't believe that all of this was really happening to me.

As individuals came into my office after our group meeting to ask about my health, I directed them to their file folder where I routinely left them messages. It seemed odd to write it out rather than simply tell them, but I had a fear of becoming hysterical if I had to say it too many times. There were a few special people who I had the nerve to tell face to face. Whether a person read it on paper and then entered my office or heard the words stuttered from my lips, the response was the same. Tears. Shock. Without exception each person was stunned that I was able to conduct the meeting I had just held without showing a hint of what I knew. This reinforced my feeling that I was a strong person—stronger, perhaps, than I had ever realized. But I knew that I *was* from good stock and that what I had just done would have been expected and not a surprise to my folks at all. I had other meetings that afternoon; one of them was with Tim. I informed him of my news. His concern for me was visible on his face. He asked if it was all right if he told Chip of my situation; I said yes. Chip, or Dr. Moses, was my other boss.

My mother had called my work, which was very rare. It's long distance and she only calls when there is a crisis. She left a message on my answering machine that Al had called her with the news from Dr. Yeo about my surgery. At the end of the day I called her back to let her know that I was okay, that somehow we'd get through this. I realized then I still needed to convince myself before I would be able to convince her of this.

Her worries and fears could be heard in the sound of her voice. "Tell me what to do. I don't know what to do to help stop all of this," she said. There was nothing that she could do to stop it. It *was* what it *was!* I am reminded of the serenity prayer. *God grant me the serenity to accept the things I cannot change, the courage to change the things I can, and the wisdom to know the difference.* These are very wise words, but sometimes hard to follow. She knew that she had no control over the fact that I had cancer. Despite her wisdom, she struggled to gain control over it. This was the first time my mother had not been the pillar of strength in our family. Our family had been through many other crises—a house fire, a barn fire, the devastating loss of all of the crops one year, other serious illnesses, the deaths of loved ones—

and she had always been the strong one. But somehow this medical crisis engulfed her in a way that made it nearly impossible to cope. I worried about her. How could I shelter her from this pain? My intent was to find comfort from her, but for a while that would not be possible, because she needed the comfort as much if not more than I.

When I left work that day and reached my car, tears flowed from me like a river. Again I turned the radio up loud, the music blaring the whole way home. My mind was no longer distracted with meetings, business calls, and memos; it was totally focused on me—my life. My mind was full of unanswerable questions. I felt angry too. Why me? What had I done to deserve this raw deal? Had I taken the wrong fork in the road somewhere and didn't know it? The last year had been a very difficult year for me. After suffering many months of stress, I spiraled into an acute depression that caused me to seek professional help. I was in an awful pit of doom and gloom. It took a lot of hard work and help from family, friends, and a good psychotherapist to pull me out of that pit. This was to be my year to celebrate life, to have a great summer, and what happens? I get told that I have cancer and need to have my breast taken off. Why? What had I done to deserve such a punishment? At least I *felt* like I was being punished.

I remember in elementary school boys would say, "I heard somebody say that if you play with yourself, your thing will fall off. Do you think that it's true?" I didn't know. I sure was glad I wasn't a boy, though. I used to wonder whether, if a girl touched her nipples a lot, they would fall off too. I made sure never to do that. As I drove home in the car that night, I thought irrational things like, "Maybe as a child I fiddled with my nipples while I was asleep and now I'm being punished by the booby demon."

When I got home, I felt exhausted. I don't think I could have felt any worse if someone had pulled me through a keyhole.

Chapter 5

It was hard for me to picture telling Laura that her mother had breast cancer and had to have her breast removed. I knew, though, that trying to protect her from the inevitable news was not the way to go. Laura was a smart twelve-year-old. She and I had always been close and she could read me like a book. She was already suspicious that something was being kept from her and it was only a matter of time before she would overhear Al and me discussing it or, worse, hear it from someone else. I decided to tell her that night. It was consoling to me that it was summer and that she wasn't in the midst of a school year. It would be hard enough for her to deal with this news without the additional burden of keeping up her grades. I decided to wait until late evening.

When I was changing my clothes, I asked her to come into the bedroom and talk with me for a while. She stretched across the bed in her favorite position and said, "So, Mom, what do you want to talk about?"

I didn't really know how to say it. Even though I had rehearsed how I would tell her and what words I would say, I looked at her face and my mind drew a blank.

"I can tell that something is the matter. There's been too much whispering around here," she said.

"Yes, there has been a lot of whispering, I guess. Remember when I came home the other night and you kept asking me what was the matter with me? Well, I didn't want to worry you then because I didn't have enough information, enough facts. But since then I've gotten more information and I'm ready to talk with you about it." She sat up on the bed and looked very concerned. "Laura, you know that I had some surgery done on my breast a week and a half ago. It was a special test to see if what was seen on my mam‑mogram pictures was anything to worry about or not. Well, the tests results are finished now. Lots of different doctors, very good doctors, have looked at them and have talked with me. The test consisted of taking some of the tissue out of my breast and looking at it under a microscope. When the doctors looked at it closely, they saw cancer cells in it. I will be having my breast taken off to get rid of the cancer that's there. The surgery is called a mastectomy, and I will be hav‑ing this mastectomy done in a few weeks."

She looked dumbfounded. She also looked confused. "How will the doctor take it off?" she asked. I explained that I would be put to sleep and the doctor would make a cut across the top of my chest and underneath my breast and remove all of the breast as well as some tissue and lymph nodes under my arm. As I've mentioned before, Laura doesn't like to see blood, needles, or anything that implies pain. Usually she puts her hand up to her mouth and says, "Don't talk about it. I'll faint." But this time she didn't. Her curiosity was too high and she wanted to understand exactly what I was talking about.

Breasts have always been a special focal point for Laura. She worried throughout her tenth and eleventh year of life that she wouldn't have big breasts. It was plain to see by the amount of peer pressure she was getting at school that this was a major worry in her life. "What if they don't grow? I'll be a freak. None of the boys will like me. I want big boobs like you have. What if it skips a generation and I have boobs like Grandma? That would make me feel awful because everybody is growing big ones in school but me." Heavens. The things that we worry about in youth. My grandmother has large breasts but my mother is a very tiny woman (size two). I, however, have large breasts like my grandmother, so I could see why Laura would make the correlation that this special big-boob gene might have skipped her generation. The kids were so fixated about this issue that I wouldn't have been surprised to see it listed as a subject on her report card. It could say, "Laura Shockney—boob class. Grade: D (comments from instructor: needs improvement. Not progressing as expected.)"

As a matter of fact, when Laura was only three years old she was fixated on breasts. She loved to play dress up and enjoyed wearing my jewelry. My mother had even made her a little lab coat that she wore to make believe that she was "a nurse like Mommy." Over the winter months that year I noticed that Laura's nipples were very red and she complained that her chest hurt her. After about five days of her complaining at night when I put her to bed, with her nipples persistently red and inflamed, I called our pediatrician. He agreed to see her the next morning.

I took the day off to take her for her appointment. I thought that maybe this was some kind of infection. Mastitis? I was familiar with mastitis having lived on a dairy farm. I also had personally experienced it after Laura was born. I developed a breast abscess which subsequently progressed into mastitis, which was very painful. Now my poor baby might have it. I felt awful for her.

She sat out in the waiting room with me, holding my hand very tightly. She didn't like going to the pediatrician. Though he was always very nice and I felt he was really great with kids, she associated him with "needle shots" and would have been thrilled never to lay eyes on his face for the rest of her life. Finally it was our turn and we went into the exam room.

"Laura, your mommy says that your chest doesn't feel good. Let me see your chest," the doctor said. Laura reluctantly lifted up her shirt but showed a facial expression of displeasure. He looked at her nipples closely and pressed around them to feel for lumps.

"So you say she has been complaining when it's time to go to bed that her nipples hurt? And that's been going on for about five days?" I confirmed this information with a nod. "Well I don't think that it's mastitis. I don't think that it's an infection at all, but I think that it can be easily cured." Great, I thought. So what is it? He turned to Laura and said, "Laura, have you been touching you chest, your nipples, a lot?" the doctor asked.

I was stunned by such an inquiry. But not as shocked as I was with the response from my child. "Yes. I been pulling on them to help make them grow so I can look like Mommy." If I had false teeth in my head, they would have clappered right on out and onto the floor at this point.

The doctor said, "Well, that's what I thought. It would be best if you didn't pull on them so hard. That's why your chest hurts at night. You eat lots of vegetables and they'll grow all by themselves." Then he turned to me and said, "Well, now we know the cause and the solution." It cost me thirty-eight dollars to learn that my child had been pulling on her nipples. You can bet your bottom dollar that the next time Laura had anything other than a true medical condition like chicken pox or strep throat, I quizzed her thoroughly before venturing back to the pediatrician.

As you can see, breasts have been a priority with my child for a long time.

I sat beside Laura on our bed and looked at her beautiful green eyes. She had a look of anxiety as well as an expression of inquisitiveness, because I had told her I was going to be losing part of my body to cancer. Her first question was, "Are you going to die?" I told her that I didn't think so, that God was the only one who knew when any of us were going to die, but I had no plans of doing so anytime soon. I explained that I had excellent doctors and the cancer had been caught early. Then she asked me some surprising questions.

"Will they let you bring your breast home with you from the hospital? After all, it is yours. They have no right to keep it." This was something I didn't expect to be asked. I explained to her that I would not be bringing it home with me because I had no need to keep it and the doctors would be doing lots of tests on it to analyze the tissue in it. It made me choke up a little when I pictured in my mind exactly how the pathology department did these tests. Someone slicing it up like a deli clerk who had just received a request for three pounds of thinly sliced ham was an unpleasant image.

Then she asked me if the doctor would take my right breast and move it to the middle of my chest. Now that was an interesting image. Definitely not your average feminine figure. When I asked her why she would think this, she said that she was afraid I would look funny with a breast only on one side and that I'd probably lean to the right when I walked. I told her I would not be having the remaining breast relocated and instead I would have an artificial breast that I would wear in my bra on the left side to replace the one that the doctor would take away.

Then I took her into the living room and showed her in the Sears catalog what a breast prosthesis looked like and what the mastectomy bras looked like. She was quite intrigued. She especially liked the idea of having a pocket in the bra to put the prosthesis in. I told her the story about Miss Bertha losing her prosthesis on the tenth hole of the golf course because her bra didn't have a pocket. She said, "Well, that pocket can be used for other things, too, Mom. When you go to the ATM, you can put your money in the pocket and that way nobody could steal it." Yes, I thought, it was definitely a unique idea. I'm not sure that I'd send it into *Woman's Day* magazine as the "helpful hint of the month," but it was definitely something to keep in mind for future reference.

I encouraged her to ask me questions as she thought of them and to let me know what worried her about the experience that our family was going through. I also told her that "Mommy would look different," but I didn't elaborate on that point. We would have many opportunities to talk more about all of this. I told her that I felt very sad about having to have this surgery and there would be times that I would cry. I told her to just give me a hug and kiss and let me cry. I needed to cry and that was good for me to get those feelings out of my system.

Laura went to bed shortly after our talk. When I kissed her good night she looked to me like she did when she was three—tiny, fragile, and oh so special to me. I gave her a kiss on the cheek called a bumble bee kiss like I used to when she was very small, and she squeezed me tightly.

Al and I sat outside on the deck that night and I recapped the conversation I had with Laura. He looked amazed as I told him the questions that were the real stumpers for me. We started to develop black humor that night and I realized just how powerful laughter and especially black humor could be. We talked about what a conversation piece my breast would be sitting on the mantle above the fireplace in a large jar. When our friends came over, we could say, "Now here is Al's deer that he shot two years ago on the Eastern shore. Doesn't it have a magnificent rack? Over here is the fifty-inch blue fish he caught in the Chesapeake Bay last summer. And, oh yes, this is Lillie's left breast. Isn't it lovely?"

We also talked a lot about how fixated society is on breasts. The bigger the better. I told him that recently one of the construction workers working near the hospital had whistled at me; I was sure this guy was probably a boob man. I was wearing a cashmere sweater that particular day. I told Al, "Well, after the surgery, if that guy is out there and whistles at me again, I'll yell over to him that he's only half right now!" We also joked about other things. "Gee, there has got to be an easier way to lose weight than this method. I guess I'll be leaving the hospital about five pounds lighter. Al got a big charge out of Laura's suggestion that I hide the money I withdraw from the ATM. Well, it would definitely be a safe place to keep it, but I don't know what the reaction would be when I pulled the money out to pay a bill. Can you picture me in the grocery store? The cashier would ring up the bill and I'd go rooting for my money. By the time I got the cash out of my bra, either the police would be there to arrest me for indecent exposure or the store would be empty due to people screaming and running for their lives!

Al was very sensitive and clever. He rarely said the humorous quips himself. He let me do that. It was far better to have me be the jokester than for him to say something and possibly catch me at a bad time when I wouldn't find it so funny. He was very happy to hear me tell these funny stories, though, and knew that it was good for me. And it was good for him. Laughter was like a special tonic. It lifted our spirits and kept us thinking in a positive way. It still does.

Chapter 6

I gave Al the unpleasant assignment of calling his family and telling them the bad news. His mother was very concerned and emotional about it. Al's older brother, Jack, had lost his wife due to cancer of the colon and liver; my mother-in-law feared I'd be the next daughter-in-law to go. Jack, himself, was very struck by it. After his wife's death he moved to a neighborhood not far from ours and routinely spent a lot of time with us. Just as he was piecing his life back together, he was delivered all too familiar news. Al's younger brother, Denny, just couldn't believe it. My age and the fact that I've never smoked or drunk or done other things known to cause cancer left him perplexed.

It was going to be several weeks before my surgery was done. I had asked if it was possible to give me this extra time so I could get things organized at work prior to my surgery date. My job is a stressful and hectic one. Dealing with issues about the quality of medical care and problems for patients related to insurance companies not covering bills creates a lot of tension.

However, working at the Hopkins Hospital reduced a lot of uneasiness. I knew I had access to the best medical care in the country. I feel bad for patients who have to travel blindly through today's health care system, having to figure out if they are receiving good care and trying to decipher where and how to get medical advice. It must be very hard and extremely nerve racking, particularly when a patient is in a life-threatening situation. Time is of the essence and choosing the wrong doctor or treatment can be a fatal error.

When I went to work the next day, I was approached by other members of my staff regarding the status of my biopsy results. A lot of tears flowed over the next few days, both from me and the folks who worked for me.

I wanted to not have this medical crisis disrupt my ability to be productive and get on with my daily activities. Each day I'd tell myself, "Just do it." Maybe if I had taken off my high heels and put on Nikes and a jogging suit it would have been easier. Of course, then people would have thought this health care executive was in need of a psychiatric consultation, and they might have been right! Over the next few days my office became a combination Hallmark store and florist shop. It made me feel good that so many people cared about me.

I mentioned to a friend that it had only been a few months back that I was eating lunch with a group from my department and we were discussing the recent death of the vice-president of nursing service at the hospital. She had died of breast cancer and it shocked every employee who knew her. It seemed ironic that she had been an oncology nurse for many years prior to being promoted to her position. People at the lunch table that day were dumbfounded. I spoke the words of doom to the group. "Breast cancer doesn't single out a particular type of person; it doesn't exclude any race. It doesn't focus in on people of a specific profession. It does not discriminate. It is a serious concern, or at least should be, for all women. There are twenty-eight women in our department. That means that if the statistics remain unaltered, three of us will probably develop breast cancer sometime in our lifetimes." I must have looked like the ghost of Christmas yet to come. The women looked at me in horror, as if I knew which three it would be. Little did I know that the countdown to identifying the first of the three would be known to us so soon.

That particular week quite a few of the staff who were over forty years old called their doctors to get booked for a mammogram. Anyone who hadn't gotten a mammogram then definitely signed up for one when they heard I had been drafted as the first member of our department to be enrolled in the breast cancer survivor club. I called my radiologist friend and told him the outcome of my breast biopsy and suggested that if the radiology department wanted to have a two-for-one sale on mammogram pictures that this was the week to offer it. He too was surprised by my news. Despite the appearance of the microcalcifations, what was hoped and believed to be benign was not.

It was hard for me to decide whether to tell others at the hospital that I had breast cancer. I, at first, didn't want people to know other than my own staff. Then I gave more thought to it and talked with Al about it and we decided that the more emotional support I had, the better off I would be. Plus I needed to explain to people why I would be moving my schedule around as well as why other staff from my department would be attending meetings for me. I wasn't prepared for the reactions of some folks, though. There were times I wasn't really sure who was supporting and consoling whom. There were those (mostly other nurses) who hugged me and showed their support and offered whatever would be helpful to me whether I was at the hospital or at home. There were other folks who fell into tears and needed consoling themselves. It definitely made me aware of the vast number of people who associated this diagnosis with death. The recent death of our VP had probably fostered these beliefs. Then there were people who had heard it through the hospital grapevine that I was "sick." These poor unknowing souls were caught completely off guard. One of them said to me, "I heard that you were sick and were going to be in the hospital, but that must have been a false rumor because you look great—healthy as a horse!" When I responded by saying that the rumor wasn't all misinformation and that I was scheduled for a mastectomy, he said, "It's got to be a mistake. The doctor has made a mistake, Lillie, because you look fine."

Well, yes, it was true. I did look fine. Of course, most women who are diagnosed with breast cancer look fine. I would imagine that even if I had been diagnosed in a much later stage of the disease, I probably would have looked peachy keen.

I wondered what people, particularly those who didn't have a medical background, thought someone with breast cancer should look like. Perhaps her bra would have a neon sign that would glow through her blouse and say, "I'm sick and am going to be amputated soon." Maybe the affected breast would blow up twice the size of its mate and that would be a clue that something was wrong.

Of course this misconception that breast cancer is a visible illness is why it is necessary to do self breast exams and why mammography is so valuable. This disease is subtle during its initial phases of establishing residency in a woman's breast. It usually moves in quietly and without any fanfare—no trumpets blaring, no fever, no edema, no pain. It operates on squatter's rights and takes over whatever territory it pleases and, if left unattended, it can take over all of you.

I wanted my coworkers and others at the hospital to know the facts. I hoped that by sharing with them this very personal crisis I could gain the emotional support I needed to weather this fierce storm. I also hoped that I could bring *reality* to the forefront and let people know that breast cancer could happen to anyone. I hoped that by being an example of this reality, I could inspire others to seek preventive medical care for themselves and their loved ones.

There was one gentleman who I had at least monthly contact with in meetings and a fair amount of business that we handled together on the phone on a weekly basis. He came by to see me when he heard the news. His concern for me was genuine and still is. However, he had a major problem expressing it. As my husband would say, he had his tongue on top of his eye teeth and he couldn't see what he was saying. The conversation went like this: "Lillie, I'm so sorry to hear about your bad news. How are you? (He then glanced down at my chest.) They look okay. I mean that you look okay. I've always thought that they looked good. I mean that I've always thought that you looked good—healthy I mean. Are you going to be okay? Are they going to go away? I mean, are you going to come back after your mastectomy?" The poor man…his eyes were fixed on my breasts and he couldn't get his eyes to come up to mine. The harder he tried, the worse it got. I broke into hysterics. I gave him a big hug and told him that I was going to be okay. One of my breasts would go away and be replaced with a prosthetic one. The other would still be around as far as I knew. He apologized for not being able to say what he wanted to say. I told him that I really preferred the version that came out of his mouth anyway; it lifted my spirits.

There was one person whom we felt it was best to not tell over the phone or through someone else's voice. That was my grandmother. She was in her eighties and we didn't feel that it would be wise to call her as we had other family members. I knew that this would be a shock to her and we didn't want her to be more worried than was necessary. My grandfather had died just a few years before from prostate cancer. My great-grandfather had also died of the same. Both died in the house where she currently lived and she had been their caretaker till the end. Her association with cancer for the most part had been that cancer equals death. It would be important to dispel this image now. So Al decided to pay her a visit while I was at work that day. He told her what the situation was and emphasized that I would be fine, that I was going to be a survivor in the end. She took in every word.

She believed what he said. Whether she believed it because of the way that he said it or because she knew deep in her bones that it would be so, she believed, and that was all that mattered.

It was interesting to learn later that my mother had spoken to her on the phone before Al arrived at her house that day. My mother had told her the verdict and grandmother, though upset to hear the news, remained convinced that I was going to be all right. I think she had to convince my mother of this, curiously enough. Mom at this point was not dealing well with the situation. The fear of potentially losing me had overwhelmed her. The anxiety of having me undergo this kind of surgery gave her a migraine headache that would not go away.

Shirley and Jim are very dear friends of ours and have been for over fifteen years. They stopped by to see us the evening after Al spoke to them on the phone. The four of us have helped each other through various and sundry crises. Each of us has had a turn. I was now up to bat and they wanted me to know that they were there for me—and for Al. Shirley is a nurse; she knew that I was aware of what the surgery entailed and what other treatment might be lurking around the bend for me depending on the outcome of my next pathology report from surgery.

If ever you need a good cry, Shirley is a great friend to call. Having friends like her was very important to me. All too often in the past I would have closed people out of my life when the chips were down. This time, with my husband's encouragement, I wasn't going to do this. I was in a war with cancer and I needed as many people on my side as feasibly possible.

A key individual I silently turned to, in my own way, was God. I'm not the kind of person to run to church, drop on my knees, and say, "Take this away from me, please. Give me something else that I can deal with, because I can't deal with this." I do pray, however, usually at night, particularly when I'm restless and can't sleep. The house is quiet. The bedroom is dark. My thoughts are directed to my family, myself, the people I love. Just as there is an old cliché, "Be careful what you wish for," so I believe is the case with prayer. Be careful what you pray for. Though I wondered why this had happened to me, I didn't ask God to answer that. I did ask him to let me live, to be a survivor of this medical experience, because I felt that I had more responsibilities and duties to be fulfilled here on earth. I also hoped that I was worthy of having the opportunity to have more pleasures from this world. That would certainly be his decision, but I put in the request just the same. One thing I knew, though: this experience with breast cancer would change me for the rest of my life—not just physically but spiritually and emotionally as well. Becoming a club member changes a person. No longer would I say "ho hum" when someone said to me that it was important to stop and smell the roses or that today is the first day of the rest of my life. I believe these sayings were written by club members who came before me. Their words now had a very personal and profound meaning for me.

On Saturday of that week I was visited by another dear friend named Lynda. Lynda and her husband Charles have known us for a very long time. They've actually known my husband for more than twenty-five years and I've known them for about fifteen of those myself. Lynda often calls me about various problems she has. Some related to the kids, some to work, some to other family crises. I'd lend an ear and try to help get her through hard times with whatever support I could offer. I was always hesitant about reciprocating, though. For some reason I never wanted to bother anybody. My troubles were mine and not for others to have to worry about. Al had spoken to Lynda and Charles, though, and Lynda took time from her hectic schedule of housecleaning chores, baby-sitting grandchildren, and fixing meals to spend the day with me. She was a powerful dose of spiritual medicine that day. Probably more so than she will ever really know.

It is hard for me to describe Lynda to others. Anyone who has met her knows though that she is unique. In some respects, she is like a naive girl, still learning about the world. In other ways, she is very wise. One thing that you can count on is that Lynda tells it like it is and asks it like it is too! She was on a special mission that day. Her mission was to get my spirits up and keep them there. She wanted me to erase from my mind all negative thoughts. She would accept nothing else. When she arrived I was definitely gloomy and four hours later I too was convinced that I'd be okay—better than okay. I'd turn this awful experience into something positive. How? Well, again, you don't know Lynda; if you did, the question would never even pop up in your mind.

Lynda took me to the Harryman House, a restaurant only a few blocks away. We had a girl's lunch—something that rarely happened for either one of us. She told me about what was on her mind and what she had discussed with Charles the night that Al had called them with the news of my biopsy results.

"When Al called and said that it was cancer, I just couldn't believe my ears. Then he said you'd have to have a mastectomy. Oh no! But then I started thinking about it. Now let's see. What would I look like if one of my breasts were gone? So I went into the bedroom, took off my clothes, stood in front of the mirror, smashed down my left breast, and I looked at myself. Then I bent over at the waist so my breasts were dangling in the air like pendulums from a clock and tried to figure out how much my breast weighed. That's when Charles came in. He couldn't figure out what I was doing and thought that I had lost my mind or something. Then I explained that I was making believe that I was you and was trying to figure out what it would be like to have a breast gone. Well, I think that my breast weighs about three pounds. Of course I wasn't able to actually weigh it because I couldn't figure how to do that on the scale. But you know, Lillie, I think that you'll breathe better when it's gone! That breast is right over you heart and lungs, and I really do think that you'll breathe better, don't you?"

Well, as Lynda spoke and waved her hands about, describing what she had done that evening to demonstrate this science project of the hidden values of mastectomy surgery, I started laughing. I laughed and laughed until tears ran down my face. What wonderful tears they were, too—happy tears...stress-reducing tears. Lynda just looked at me, trying to figure out why I found this description so funny, which is why Lynda is Lynda. She figured that everyone would have probably done the same thing she did to simulate the experience of a mastectomy! And I'm sure there are other Lyndas out there. At least I hope so. We need more Lyndas so those of us who are going through the real experience can appreciate the humor that someone who loves us dearly can bring to the forefront.

We also had some time for more serious conversation. She was concerned about Laura's reaction to all of this. I told her that initially Laura seemed okay but a few days later she wasn't. Several nights after I had my little talk with her, I heard her crying in her room. When I went in to see what was the matter, she said she was afraid that she was the cause of my getting cancer. She said that because I had complications when she was born, maybe whatever they were had caused these cancer cells to grow. She felt totally responsible and said that if she had never been born, I would be healthy now. It really devastated me to hear those words. But I was thankful that at least she opened up and told me what was on her mind. I convinced her that her birth had nothing to do with this problem and that she was the best thing that had ever happened to me.

Lynda also wanted to reassure me that she knew that despite my concerns about my appearance, Al was going to do fine. "It's only flesh. It's not you, not the woman he married. He didn't marry you for your boobs. He loves you. And by the way, I want you to promise me you'll show me your incision after your surgery. I want to see that battle scar. And I want to see your prosthesis too. Everything!"

I took a picture of her outside on the deck, before she went home that day. We talked for four hours straight. She asked me about what worried me; I'd tell her something and then she'd have some amazing one-liner that would put it into perspective. Her real message was to not let this thing get to me. If I did, then I'd be a goner. Stay on top of it. Stay optimistic. Seek the humor in the situation whenever possible, and remember that I am loved. She agreed that God wasn't done with my stay here on earth. She put me on her prayer list and other people's prayer lists too. That was very comforting.

I had my film developed the next day at a one-hour film processing store so I could look at Lynda's face right away.

Her picture stayed strategically placed on the coffee table for me to see every evening when I got home from work.

Another family we had always been close to was the Cross family, Pat and John. Though they lived several hours away from us, we saw them quite regularly and visited together as families. Al's daughter, Roxanne (from his previous marriage), viewed them as a second set of parents. There was even a time that Roxanne lived with them, occupying an apartment they had fashioned for her in their basement when she was ready to start living more independently. Because Roxanne had married into a local family in the area where the Crosses lived, we got to see them all the more often.

Pat and John had always been healthy people in general. Of course, so had we. The same time that I was served the verdict of breast cancer, John was given the verdict of brain cancer. He and I bonded together in a very special and unique way because we were going through troubled waters simultaneously. If we were going to be in a row boat with no paddles and there was a hole in the boat, we'd gladly help each other bale.

Having two people who Roxanne was very close to be diagnosed with cancer was very traumatic for her. It was also very hard for Pat. It made us all very much aware that cancer can effect anyone, even us.

One evening when Pat and John were down visiting us, we were looking at home videos that Pat had taken at our house the previous summer. I looked at that movie and realized that these people on film laughing and telling jokes and swimming in the pool really had nothing to be laughing about. They just didn't know it yet. I was looking at myself and John, seemingly healthy on film, but both harboring cancer cells that would not make themselves known to us for several months to come.

So the resources I needed, the emotional ones at least, were quickly being rounded up. My mother was rounding up even more of them behind the scenes. Work schedules were being reviewed and assignments being prepared to be divvied up for the time I would be away from work after my surgery.

Chapter 7

My next plan of attack was to educate myself about breast cancer. Even though I was a nurse I didn't feel like an expert when it came to various kinds of breast cancer, treatment options, and research protocols that were currently in use. I wanted to be an expert, though, and fast. Over the weekend I went to the mall and ravaged the bookstores there. I purchased the book called *Dr. Love's Breast Book.* I also got a few other books on cancer treatment modalities. On Friday, prior to coming home from work, I connected up with Jean Wainstock, the breast cancer clinical nurse specialist Dr. Yeo had told me about. She was very helpful and dropped off a lot of reading material published by the American Cancer Society about breast cancer.

I got home from the bookstores and promptly started reading. I couldn't put the material down. I felt better about what was going on in my life as long as I could read about it and remove some of the mystery and confusion about my future. Definitely Dr. Love's book was the best money I had ever spent. It contained drawings as well that I was able to share with my husband that showed what the surgery would look like—an end result drawing at least. All of the information was important and the author clearly understood how I was feeling. It was as if this book were for me specifically, and about me. It gave me peace of mind. It also served as a constant reminder that many women who already were club members had gone through this experience before me. Their thoughts and feelings were merely echoes of my own in many cases.

I also felt that information was power. I could perhaps gain some control over this experience if I was well-versed about the subject. I think I could have read all night that first night I had this material in my hands. I didn't even stop to eat. My husband asked me to give my eyes a break and come to the table twice, but I couldn't. He compromised and fixed a plate for me and brought it into the living room. He, too, could see my energy level rising as I read more. He told me to mark any sections I wanted him to read, and that made me feel really good. Many times he said to me that even though he was not the one with the diagnosis, he felt the pain, anxiety, and fear. That's when I knew that we had a good marriage. If ever I had doubted it, this confirmed it for me. I could see in his face that this truly was our pain, our problem, and I knew that with his strength I could get myself up on top of this dreadful thing and be a winner, a survivor.

I also started scanning the Yellow Pages for advertisements for mastectomy supplies. I wanted to learn everything. There was no time to lose. I became intrigued with the names of shops that carried mastectomy bras, prosthesis, swimwear, and other garments. They had names like, We Fit, Perfectly You, A Special Touch, Jodee's Inner Fashions—very subtle names. It made me realize that to be an active member of this club, you had to know the code words to figure out where to shop. I phoned one of the stores listed. They had a recording on their answering machine that said they specialized in breast prosthesis for use as external reconstruction to be worn during intimate moments. I fantasized that perhaps what they sold were stick-on boobs that had a tassel hanging from a fake nipple that was battery operated. One could flick a switch and get the tassel to go clockwise, or if your husband preferred, counterclockwise. I ended up visiting their shop at a later time and was disappointed to find that their phone advertisement was referring to the creation of a breast prosthesis that was made from the mold taken from your other breast. It was very expensive too, close to sixteen hundred dollars. (I have since spoken to other club members who have purchased a prosthesis there and they love it. It was too expensive for my needs, though.) I would have preferred not to have had my fantasy shattered and wished that I had never paid them a visit. Oh well. Perhaps if Blaze Star ever has a friend who has breast cancer, she will create such a line of prosthetic gadgets and call her shop Blaze's Boobery Boutique. I might even consider stopping in there for a novelty item for a special occasion!

Al surprised me that Sunday evening and bought me crab. It was a hard decision to put my reading material down, but the smell of steamed crab did the trick. He was right. I needed a break. I had read over four hundred pages of material in two days without skimming over anything, and I had learned the material well enough to recite just about any section back to him verbatim. He won me over, though. I love steamed crabs. He told me he had enough money on him to buy me one and a half dozen roses or to buy me two dozen steamed crabs. He chose wisely; he knew me well. Crab was far more romantic to me that day than flowers ever would have been.

On Monday it was back to the old grind stone. Work was very good for me. It kept my mind off of my troubles, at least most of the time, and it made me feel productive. I realized that morning when I was in the shower that I seemed to be unconsciously avoiding touching my left breast. I'd rub the bar of Coast soap all over, except there. At first I wasn't touching it because the incision was still tender, but that was no longer the case. There was what seemed to be purposeful avoidance and even though I was aware of it, I wasn't able to do anything about it. I felt as if this part of my body weren't deserving of good hygiene. It was infected with something bad, and perhaps touching it would encourage it to spread. Even though I knew this was a silly thought, I still avoided it. I also avoided looking in mirrors when I got out of the shower. Avoidance was my defense mechanism, and I maintained it, generally speaking, until my surgery date. I didn't even bother to look at how well, or not well, my incision was healing. Why bother? It was only healing long enough to be cut off and discarded.

I wondered if, after the mastectomy, some medical student would be given my breast to examine and study the stages of tissue healing after surgery. That was about all that this incisional biopsy/lumpectomy incision was good for now.

I chuckled to myself on occasion about how upset I had been when I first came home from my outpatient surgery and saw the three-and-one-half-inch incision. To think that I was worried and distressed about how my breast looked post-op…Well, the joke was surely on me now. I realized that I should have been thrilled to have had only a three-and-one-half-inch incision that dimpled my breast inwardly. When I said my prayers that night, I learned a valuable lesson. I learned to be grateful for what I had and not wish for more than had been given to me. It was a hard pill to swallow, but a lesson that would last me a lifetime. At least I hoped it would.

The nights were hardest for me. Even after my prayers I would find myself sobbing. Al would hold me tightly. He didn't say much. That was best. No words were needed. I just couldn't believe this was happening to me. It continued to feel like a bad dream. I would tell myself that if ever I woke up and confirmed that this was all a dream, I'd never eat before bedtime again.

I decided it would be smart for me to see my psychotherapist more often between this time and my surgery date, so we had weekly sessions. She was helpful in letting me express things I was afraid to say out loud even to myself. She served as a good person to bounce information off of to make sure I really wasn't losing my mind, just my breast. Her name was Marla.

My other boss, Chip, came by for an unexpected visit during that week. Tim had told him of my situation and he wanted to show his support. It was hard for him to express his emotions, but that was okay. I had known Chip for more than a decade and what emotion he showed me that day was more than I would have ever expected. He reassured me that I was in good hands with the medical and surgical team there at the hospital. Those words weren't necessary, though; I had confidence in my doctors. But it still was nice to have it reaffirmed.

I concentrated much of my time on making short-term and long-term plans for my office—all of the what ifs, like what if I need to be out longer than a month, how should I divvy up the workload? What if there are complications and I need to be out longer or need chemotherapy? It was very important to me not to leave any loose ends. I didn't want to be a burden to anybody. I also didn't want to return to chaos.

My staff, especially Scott, Marge, Bryanna, Joyce, and Sheila, and of course Diane, were really super. "You just tell us what you want us to do and we'll do it," they said. Unfortunately, it was easier to hear those words than it was to figure out how to reallocate the work. Projects I had halfway finished I wanted to have wait until I was able to finish them myself. Decisions that needed to be made at a director's level would either have to be punted to Tim or wait for my return. It was complicated. I decided that, if it was at all possible, I would have work brought home to me after my first week or so of recuperation. So that's how we left it. Assignments were given, work flow rearranged, and a schedule prepared. It felt awkward, but very necessary just the same.

I knew I would have about two weeks or so left before I would be on vacation, then upon my return I would have surgery. My transformation surgery—the surgery that would hopefully transform me from a breast cancer victim to a breast cancer survivor. Time really raced by at work most days, but it inched itself along at night. Nights fell into a steady pattern of having dinner, reading any new material I was able to get my hands on about breast cancer and its treatment, reviewing whatever documents that I had brought home from work to complete, then to bed for a night of restless sleep. I'd get to bed and, within about twenty minutes, start crying. Al would hold me and rub my back and I'd cry. The living nightmare continued for weeks.

Chapter 8

Here it was summer and I wasn't having the time of my life as I had expected. We had planned a Hawaiian party at our house for weeks and now I was undecided if due to these new developments whether we should cancel it or not. I wanted people to have a good time. It was a party, not a funeral. But I didn't know if I could have a good time or not. I certainly didn't want to go on a crying jag right in front of everybody. The majority of the folks we had invited were people from the hospital and crying in front of them would have been very embarrassing. Instead of handing out Hawaiian leis, I would be handing out Kleenex. Not good. So we gave it a lot of careful thought. The conclusion we reached was that this party would be one of the best things we could do for ourselves. We would be surrounded by friends who were also work associates and we'd have a happy time! So the party plans stayed intact.

Because not everyone who had been invited was aware of my present health status, I decided to send out some personal notes. My mistake was that I sent these documents to their work addresses and didn't realize they were out of town and wouldn't be back at work to review their mail until after the party. My intention was to not have anyone surprised by this news in the event that someone brought it up. I did request of the attendees that people avoid the subject for the day, though. This was to be a party—a time to relax, eat, drink, swim, tell funny stories, and enjoy each other's company. Hugs were welcome. It was not to be a pity party. And it worked out great! Everyone had a good time, including me. We laughed and talked and ate until we were all ready to explode. I didn't know that several of our guests (Haya, Albert, and Earl) had not received my personal note and were unaware of the circumstances at hand. I just thought they were being polite and respectful of my request not to discuss it. But I could tell by some of their comments that they were still in the dark, particularly when they were discussing work related projects and things we would be working on together in the middle of July, which at that time was a few weeks away. I didn't listen to the detail of the projects being discussed because I knew I would be working on my own project—my project of being transformed from a cancer victim into a cancer survivor. Certainly this would be the most important project of my lifetime to date.

We had decided to invite my parents over for the party too. We wanted to visit with them, give them an opportunity to meet some of my colleagues, and see me in a happy mood. We hoped that maybe it would lift their spirits too. Dad and Mom arrived early to visit with us before the gang arrived. This was the first time that they had seen me since my diagnosis was made known to them and they needed some time alone with me. My mother aged ten years in two or three weeks. She was really having a hard time of it. I felt awful for her. I was the cause of her looking so sad, so worried, and there was nothing I could do to make it go magically away. I was careful not to succumb to the overwhelming feeling to sit with her and go on a major crying jag. But

I stayed focused on the party, the food preparation, and the necessity to have a fun day.

My father camped out alone for a while in the living room. When I finished fixing the food trays, I went in to him. Mom was occupied with Laura, catching up on who Laura's latest boyfriend was. When I entered the living room I found Dad with his eyes fixed on the open pages of *Dr. Love's Breast Book*. He looked ill. He was looking at the drawings of the mastectomy incision post-op. He looked up at me and started crying. This was a surprise to me. My dad wasn't the kind to show emotion. He always wanted to present himself as a tough guy. He really isn't, though. Looking at the book upset him. It put the problem into a very physical perspective and one that was too close for comfort for him. He didn't know what to say and was distressed that I had found him crying. I told him I was going to be okay and I wanted this to be a good day—a fun day—for everyone. He responded as he often did in family crisis. "I know that all I do is talk about money, but that is all I have to give you. If you need anything, just buy it. Your mother is going to put money in a joint account for you. Spend it. Medical bills will come in fast now. I don't want you to want for anything and go without because you don't have the money to pay for things that you need."

He was right. Dad frequently talked about money. It was a major part of his upbringing. It was a major focal point in my mother's life too. Dad, I think, associated money with security, and he wanted me to be secure. He wanted to provide me protection, even if the only protection he could give me was financial protection. He knew that money couldn't rid me of this problem, but he wanted me to have the best medical treatment that money could buy. He didn't want me to feel distracted by monthly bills if I had to be off from work for an extended period of time. He knew that I was the bread winner in the family. My husband was laid off from work several years ago on a medical disability due to a back problem. What he didn't know was that I too thought as he did, or, better said, as he and Mom had taught me. I had a lot of sick time built up, plus I had good health care insurance. I also had additional short-term and long-term disability insurance in the event of a medical problem like this. So I felt financially stable, at least for the time being. His gesture was genuine and it was his way of showing me that he wanted me well. It was also his way of saying that he loved me.

The party went off without a hitch, at least almost without a hitch. Toward the end of the day, when people were preparing to leave, I saw Haya talking with my mother. My mother looked teary eyed; I sensed that she had taken a moment to talk with Haya about her concerns about me. Haya was a physician and someone who my mother had spent time with before, so it was natural for my mother to talk with her in private that day. Shortly after their conversation, my folks left and headed back to their farm on the Eastern Shore. Haya frequently glanced over at me and smiled, but she looked perplexed. Then when she was ready to leave, she asked if she could have a word with me. We took a brief stroll down the sidewalk. She told me that my mother seemed very upset. When she had inquired what was troubling her, my mother responded by saying that she was worried about me. Worried that she would lose me. Frustrated that she couldn't control the situation. My mother hadn't explained what the situation was, however. That's when I figured out that Haya hadn't gotten my letter. She had been out of town and hadn't seen her mail yet. I paused a moment.

First I thought I'd simply tell her to wait and read her mail, then I realized that this would not have been a fair answer. I had almost gotten through the afternoon without mention of it. It felt good too. For a while, I could fantasize that it was only a dream. Here I stood before a friend who knew something strange was going on, but who had no idea what. I finally got up the nerve to tell her. "I've been diagnosed with breast cancer." Where are the Kleenex when you need them? We both burst into tears. She, like so many others, offered her support. Being a doctor herself, she instinctively began asking me medical questions about my treatment plan. She also said that she knew that neither Albert nor Earl knew about my medical problem and she offered to give them a status report of my situation.

Why was this happening to me? I used to think when I was little that God had a big book the size of my father's cow barn. In this book there were two pages for each person on Earth. On one page he wrote check marks when you did something really good; on the other side he'd mark when you were really bad. When you died, he'd add up the check marks. If the number of good check marks outnumbered the number of bad check marks, then you would have a place with him beyond the pearly gates. If you didn't though… well, you would go to a place that would be really awful and full of demons. (I guess if I had been a child of the '90s I would have had God use a calculator or computer to keep score.)

As an adult I developed different views on the subject. Perhaps God has a big matrix chart on each person, divided up into various categories that include good experiences and bad experiences. He assigns a grade to our performance with each experience. For example, if you have a good experience like having a baby, he evaluates your performance as a mother. Were you loving, kind, caring, nurturing, and so forth? But, I wonder, if you are diagnosed with breast cancer, then what is his criterion for measuring performance? Does he evaluate how well we deal with body disfigurement? Is it perhaps a test of marriage vows, about the "for better, for worse, in sickness and in health" part?

Well, if so, I wanted to get a good score. I wanted to stay on top of this thing and not let it get me. I wanted him to see that I had faith and could deal with it, no matter what the long-term outcome would be. This was just a piece of flesh and not really me—not my mind and certainly not my soul. My goal was to be a breast cancer survivor, and to become one I would do whatever was asked of me. I wanted to get an A+ in this matrix box.

Chapter 9

On Father's Day, we called Dad. Unfortunately, Dad was out. Mom was home by herself and was having, as she termed, "a bad day." She had apparently been crying before she even heard my voice on the phone. She kept saying that she wanted a miracle and had contacted many churches to ask that my name be placed on their prayer lists. She wanted to reach someone who knew about Mother Seton, the saint from Maryland. She was very upset and perhaps angry—distressed that she had no control over what was happening to her child. Feeling helpless, wanting a miracle to occur that would rid me of this awful thing, she could not be comforted by anything I said.

I felt awful for her and for myself. I tried to reassure her that I would be all right, but she just couldn't accept that as an answer. She kept telling me that this wasn't supposed to be happening to me. I had had enough things go wrong in my life. She wanted it to be her. She told me that if this were her breast, she'd feel okay about it. She could deal with that. I told her repeatedly that it was not her choice and it wasn't her fault. No one had pulled my name out of a hat and said I won the booby prize. I also told her I felt relieved that it was I who had it, because, of the two of us, I was in better physical and emotional health. Al also tried to comfort her, but it seemed useless. This was a woman who would walk through fire for her family, but this time there was no fire to walk through to take the problem away…to remove the hurt and emotional pain.

My mother has always been a very active member of her Episcopal church, perhaps even recognized as a pillar of the church, yet she was not receiving the peace of mind she so desperately needed at this moment in her life. Her insistence to contact Mother Seton surprised me, because we're not even Catholic. I started thinking that perhaps much of the problem was that she may have felt trapped somehow—trapped between two generations that had been stricken with cancer. Her father died of prostate cancer. His death was a very painful experience for her. She and I stood together at his bedside in her parents' home when he took in his last breaths. He was alert until the end and did not want to die. His life was extended by a few days because of her presence, I believe. He wanted to be with her and fought off the closing of death's door for as long as he could. Now she was looking at the generation behind her, her own child, and feared that she would once again be placed in a situation that was all too familiar. Her fear of its potential threat overwhelmed her and challenged her to gain control in any way that she could. Prayer was a very constructive way and I was glad that she sought that path. It felt reassuring to know after that day that when I went to bed at night there were many people across the state of Maryland and even in nearby states who were asking God to take care of me (and perhaps grade me on a curve).

I spend a lot of time on weekends running errands and shopping. Shopping malls started to take on a different image for me, though. I started doing what I remember my brother doing as a teenager when he and I would go shopping somewhere—I started looking at women's breasts. I felt compelled to. I would look at each woman I would see and try to pick out experienced members of the club. I'd look to see if their breasts bounced when they walked. If they did, then I assumed that theirs were real and that they weren't in the breast cancer survivor club. Then I would look at people and think that they might be future recruits into the club. Since one in nine women becomes affected sometime in her life by breast cancer, then I could hypothetically calculate who might be a future draftee. I'd count the women as they'd walk by . . . one, two, three, four, five, six, seven, eight, *nine!* Oh no! She might be the next one. And she probably doesn't even know it. Oh, the poor dear. No matter how many women I saw or where I saw them, I wondered if I was secretly in the presence of a post-mastectomy patient. It was really nutty, but that's what I did.

Poor Al. When he was with me I'd ask for his opinion too. "What do you think of that set over there? The one on the right doesn't seem to bounce as much as the one on the left. Do you agree?" He'd just shrug his shoulders and walk on down the aisles with me. Clearly I should have had my brother with me, because he was a real boob man. He'd know the answers for sure, but he lived in Japan.

Sometimes, when Laura and I were at a mall or in the grocery store together, I'd ask her to help me locate a woman who might be wearing a fake boob. Clearly, she didn't want to play this game at all. She would usually walk the other direction. Perhaps she was afraid of what I would do if I was successful in my search. Maybe she thought I would ask to touch someone's breast or something. I never did find one. Despite my routine explorations, I came up empty-handed and was convinced that if there were others who had had a mastectomy, then all of them must have had reconstruction.

Though arrangements had been made for me through the hospital for a Reach to Recovery volunteer to see me after my surgery, I longed to talk to someone now, before the deed was done. I called the Reach to Recovery office and requested to speak with a breast cancer survivor who had had a mastectomy, was under the age of forty, and was married. It was clear to me that they were not used to receiving calls directly from patients and that they usually don't connect volunteers up with anyone until the patients are in a post-op state. But I wanted to talk to someone about what I should expect upon waking up, and about other personal matters like intimacy with a mate, and I wanted to talk *now*, not two weeks from now. In two weeks I would be able to answer most of the questions that were burning in my mind by doing a personal self-evaluation of my own recovery room experience. So the woman who answered the phone agreed to have a volunteer call me back. I also requested that the volunteer be a large-busted woman. I felt that talking to a woman who wore a size 32 AA bra before her surgery was not in the same boat with me, who wore a 42 D cup. That was an important variable in my book.

Two days later, I received a call from a volunteer. She was helpful, but I didn't feel as connected to her emotionally as I had hoped to be. She was a 34 A.

I also had a major concern about some other medical issues that related to my care and treatment. These issues surrounded the kind of anesthesia I would be receiving. I had a history of problems receiving general anesthesia in the past. At the age of thirteen, I had had an emergency appendectomy and had intraoperative complications from anesthesia. My blood pressure bottomed out and my recovery time in the recovery room was extended by three hours as a result. When I was in labor with Laura and a vaginal delivery attempt was unsuccessful, an emergency C-section was done. I demanded not to be put to sleep because of my reaction to general anesthesia, so a rapid spinal anesthesia was given. Unfortunately, I had trouble with it as well and awoke in an ICU due to respiratory failure. This pattern repeated itself again after I had surgery for abdominal adhesions and ovarian cyst removal. Needless to say, the thought of general anesthesia concerned me. I didn't want to die. I tried to figure out what I could do to influence the odds in my favor. I decided to ask Tim if he could connect me up with an appropriate physician who could look out for me during this surgery.

One thing in my favor was that I was having the surgery in a controlled environment. What I mean by that is that I wasn't having this procedure done as an emergency operation like a gunshot wound patient does. Each time I had experienced trouble before, it was during and immediately following emergency surgery. Another advantage was that I was in a position to make a special request for a particular anesthesiologist. I'm sure all of them were excellent, but again, I was seeking control. Tim offered to tell chief of the department of anesthesiology about my medical history. I was unable to get any of my medical records from previous hospitalizations, so he had to explain based on my memory. It would have been best to have the records so they could see what drugs I had been given, but that was not possible. I asked Tim to ask the following question of the chief of the Sandmen Gang: "If I were the chief's wife and, assuming he loves his wife, whom would he recommend to put her to sleep, knowing this specific medical history with anesthetic agents?" He did ask. The answer given back to him was Dr. Charles Beattie.

Dr. Beattie called me that same day and introduced himself. He reviewed my medical history, surgical/anesthetic events, and what kind of allergies I have. Since the last time I had surgery (ten years before), many new and improved drugs were on the market and being used with some of the more standard anesthesia agents. He arranged for me to be examined and for chest x-rays and some other tests to be done, including some special views of my neck because it was part of my medical history that I had a narrow airway. Dr. Beattie (Charlie) was wonderful. I could tell by his voice and the depth of his medical evaluation that I was in excellent hands. Anesthesia was still a worry, but not as severe of one as it had been, in my mind.

As the days grew nearer, Laura started spending more time with me rather than in her room, listening to her cassette tapes blaring. We'd watch a funny movie or play *Wheel of Fortune* on the computer. It was clear that her concerns for my survival and well-being were resting heavily on her mind. I heard "I love you, Mommy" at least six times a day. "Even though you say that you will be different after your surgery, I don't think you'll change. You'll be the same to me."

Al also tried to provide me constant reassurance that he would still love me. My breast being gone wouldn't make a bit of difference to him. He kept telling me this, especially at night when we were in bed. He kept saying it, but I was afraid to believe it. "You don't understand yet what my incision is going to look like. You can't tell me that it won't make a difference until you see it. Then we'll both see how you feel." I also told him that it could be months before I would let him even see my incision. He said that would be my decision, but I was worrying about nothing. He said he respected my wishes. "After all," he said, "you've never seen me without my teeth in. I'm funny about that, you know." We chuckled about that. We'd been married almost fifteen years and in all that time I had never seen him without his upper plate in. He slept with his upper plate in, too. I told him that maybe I'd make a deal with him. He could show me his toothless smile and I'd show him my one-breasted chest. He thought that that seemed like a fair deal. I reminded him that he needn't worry about having to practice his smile for a while because I didn't think that I'd be ready for several weeks after my surgery, possibly even several months. He told me he'd wait for the signal from me.

Chapter 10

During the last week of June, my brother, his wife, and two his children came to visit us. They had come home from Japan for vacation. Robert, Mary, and the kids (Julie age eleven, and David age seven) had been in Japan for nearly three years. He was a colonel in the air force—one of those F-16 pilots who like to travel through the air like their hair was on fire. Robert's family hadn't been home for a year. Their visit with us was a strained one because of my health. When I was diagnosed, I couldn't even talk with them on the phone. Just to hear Robert's voice ask me, "How are you doing, Sis?" completely disintegrated me to tears. I practiced talking about my surgery a lot before they actually came. By the time they were here, I was able to discuss it as if it were happening to someone else. Robert didn't directly ask me about my health. Mary did most of the questioning. Mary's mother also had breast cancer. Her folks lived in Colorado and they would be stopping to see them after their visit with us and my parents on the farm.

We spent our time together swimming in the pool, eating crab, and watching our children play together. This was a special time to see the value of a close family unit. Lots of pictures were taken. Robert didn't need to say much to me. It wasn't necessary, and he doesn't want to dwell on sad situations. I knew his concern was genuine. Often when he visited we'd talk very little. Robert and I did discuss our family's history of having growths in some of our throats. Both Mom and I had been diagnosed and treated for these throat problems. These growths are believed possibly to be caused by exposure to strong chemicals. The link for our family was the pesticides and insecticides that Dad had used for years on the crops. Apparently they were similar to the Agent Orange used in the Vietnam War. We were all thankful that we didn't have children who were born with birth defects. It did raise the question as to whether this was a contributor to my present condition.

My father was very sentimental with Rob and his family during the visit. He had sent a personal letter in the mail to me about ten days before Rob arrived. This was a rare thing for Dad to do. It was filled with words of love and emotion. I was surprised and impressed that he mentioned the letter to Rob and Mary while we were eating our crab. He was definitely wanting to make sure that the things that had been left unsaid in the past were said now and said often. From that day on, whenever I saw Dad, he was always sure to tell me that he loved me. It was the beginning of a new relationship with him and it felt good. Our relationship had become closer because of my body betraying me and flirting with death. God truly did bring some positive moments into a very bad experience. These moments would not be fleeting, either. They would be moments that would last a lifetime . . .

for the rest of my life. Our family's goal was for that time to be a very long one.

Two days after Robert and Mary left our home, we were on a plane for vacation. Laura went with Robert to the farm to visit with her cousins. Though our vacation had been planned for months, my enthusiasm was gone about making the trip. We were to go to one of my very favorite places—Maine. I had planned to stuff myself with lobster until I couldn't stand looking at those big red crustaceans anymore. But I just didn't feel like it. My problem was that I knew that when we came home it would be time . . . time for my mastectomy to be done. I wanted to trade in our plane tickets for one-way ones and just stay there—just sit by the ocean and listen to the waves crashing and the lighthouse horn sounding in the distance. I again felt like Dorothy in *The Wizard of Oz*. The hourglass had been turned over and my time was running out. I wondered if I would feel better if I bought a pair of red sequined shoes. Probably not. Like Dorothy, I wouldn't know how to make them work anyway. And they'd be expensive and probably not on sale.

I decided to do all of my packing at once and get it out of the way. One suitcase was packed for Maine, one small bag for the hospital. I also switched my watch that day from my left wrist to my right. You may think this was an odd thing to do, but I knew that after my surgery it would need to be on the right side. That's because I'd be having a left-sided mastectomy. Some of the lymph nodes would be removed from the left armpit area (axilla) in the procedure. This results in arm edema. Some people keep the edema for a long time. Some people have experienced swelling of the arm after doing any kind of strenuous activity. It is unwise to wear anything that is constricting on the arm that is affected by the surgery. So I decided that I might as well start getting used to wearing it on the other wrist now; that way there would be one less adjustment for the future. Unfortunately, every time I'd look at my left wrist to check the time and realize I had switched it, a shroud of gloom would cover my mind. I'm a clock watcher and have been all my life, so this feeling of gloom was constant. I left the watch on its new location just the same.

We left to go to Maine as planned. On the plane I worried that I might have gotten mixed up and packed the camera in the wrong suitcase. That would have been interesting. Taking a camera into the operating room…ugh. I had placed it in the right bag after all, so it was a minor worry. I also packed my diary (which my psychotherapist friend, Marla, had recommended I keep and take with me to record my thoughts and feelings). For reading material I brought a book that was written by a breast cancer survivor. She had had a mastectomy when she was young too. I had hoped that it would be uplifting and give me a feeling of hope and support, particularly since I was now reading the last half of the book which concentrated on her life after her mastectomy had been done. It didn't uplift me at all. It made me feel worse. Here was a single woman who put into print that even after reconstructive surgery she didn't have sex for five and a half years! She wrote that men rejected her. Good heavens. What a sad thing to share with the world. I wanted to read about a woman in her thirties who had done well, physically, emotionally, and spiritually, after her surgery. This was not a woman that would serve as a role model for me. No sir. I felt sorry for her. She must have kept running into and subsequently dating some real jerks. Then I realized that I had been out of the dating game for fifteen years. I was married. It made me very thankful that I was married. It must be an awful challenge to have to date someone and make that awkward decision about when to tell him that you've had a mastectomy. "Hi. My name is Lillie. I'm a Libra. I've got one boob. What's your name?" Yes, I was among the fortunate. At least I hoped I was.

I asked myself what I would do if Al had trouble adjusting to my body after my surgery. What would he do if he couldn't adjust? He had been reassuring me that he would be fine with it. But the test had not yet come. We talked a lot about that specific issue. He hadn't seen what I would look like, so how could he possibly know that this giant scar across my chest wouldn't be a turnoff for him? I felt like taking him to a horror flick and watching his facial reactions while various grotesque monsters suddenly appeared on the screen. I also realized that I wasn't being fair to my surgeon. For all I knew, his needle work would look so good that I myself wouldn't feel offended by what I saw. But the fact of the matter was that at this moment in time I didn't know. I could only speculate.

When Al and I had private time and were in intimate situations, I usually cried—during and after. I couldn't get the thoughts out of my mind that this wonderful, loving and tender relationship was about to be abolished by a scalpel. Once I got the definitive diagnosis of breast cancer, he stopped touching me above the waist when we were in bed. I was relieved, but sometimes I misinterpreted it as his practicing no longer to touch my breasts at all. I'll still have one left, I thought to myself. Will it be off limits too because its partner was about to be evicted for demonstrating unacceptable behavior? I felt it best not to discuss it and just let time take its course in determining our future private relationship.

One evening when we were sitting out on the balcony of our room in Bar Harbor, we were talking about how long I anticipated my recovery to be. I hoped it would be about four weeks or so. I also talked to Al about a patient I had taken care of once who had had a mastectomy several years before I met her. She had been admitted for a gastrointestinal problem. She was very nice and was in her fifties at the time. I got up the nerve to ask her some questions about her breast cancer experience. She was married to a wonderful man. I had met him; it was obvious that they had a really special relationship. I asked her how long it took her to adjust to her breast being gone. Her reply was a surprising one to me. She said that on some days she didn't feel like it was gone. She had a phantom-limb sensation. Just like amputees who lose a leg or an arm, she too had the sensation that her breast was still there. She even told me that she enjoyed having her husband touch her incision in certain spots because it simulated the pleasant feeling that she used to have when her breast was still there. She absolutely shocked me when she told me that she thought that her nerve that went to her nipple was somewhere stitched in the sutures that had been sewn in her arm pit because she loved her husband to kiss her there! I know I must have looked like a very shocked and naive young woman to her that day. She said, "You might be a nurse and in your early twenties, but I can tell that you haven't had much experience in the world yet." She was right about that one. I was too embarrassed to talk with her anymore about it. Sitting in Bar Harbor seventeen years later, I would have given someone a lot of money to help me find that lady so I could talk with her again.

Al seemed very intrigued and most attentive while I was telling him this story. He didn't laugh, though I did. He told me that this could be *my* story in the near future and that I might be telling someone about our experiences yet to come. He said, "I'll nibble on your elbow, armpit, neck, anywhere!" Then, about a half-hour later, as we were going back into our room for the night, he said, "Just one question. There's no chance that your nipple nerve could end up in your rear end is there? I love you but I might have to draw the line there." We had a big laugh over that. I assured him that it would stay somewhere in the region of the incision area. I also told him that not every woman had phantom-limb sensation.

On our last night of vacation I felt well rested and much more at ease with my situation, though I must admit my mood was very unstable. The weather had not been very good for part of our trip, but we enjoyed each other's company. I appreciated the sun when it was shining and even admired the sudden changes in the weather when a thunderstorm blew in. I rarely ever had taken the time to look at the sky except when it was nice out. I was learning to value all of the weather now because it meant that I was alive. I was here. I wasn't pushing up daisies from six feet under. I was finally learning to stop and smell the roses . . .

Our last night was spent in Portland. Just as we were ready to go to bed, we decided to catch the last half of a show on TV. I don't know if it was *Prime Time Live* or *20-20* or something else, but it was great. We both needed it. The show was about a baseball player who had bone cancer that resulted eventually in the loss of his entire arm and shoulder—his pitching arm. He and his wife were both interviewed. They talked about how this tragic experience changed their lives, but in the long run for the better. Sure, he wished it had never happened to him. Sure, it resulted in his not being able to be a famous major league ball player anymore. But it strengthened their marriage; it gave them both an appreciation for life; it brought them closer to God. Now his time was spent on lecture circuits talking about his experience. He also met a lot of children who had not been as fortunate as he. These were kids who also had cancer but would eventually and in some instances swiftly be swept from this earth and taken from the people who loved them—their parents, sisters, brothers, grandparents, and friends. It gave him a new perspective about the value of life. He said that he believed God had given him this tragedy so he could instill hope into other cancer victims. Well, I didn't know whether this was so—whether God gave this to him, I mean. I do know about the other part, though, because he instilled hope in me that night. He didn't have breast cancer, but he had definitely lost a part of his body that he valued very much. He went on with his life and was clearly a better person for it. Al turned to me and said, "That will be us very soon."

Chapter 11

I went into work for just a day or so after vacation and before my surgery. I wanted to clear up any burning items that needed to be handled so I would truly feel I was starting with as clean a slate as possible when I went out for my surgical sick leave. I also had an appointment in the same-day surgery center to have a preoperative evaluation, a chest x-ray, blood work, and such. The big day was now only two days away. I also saw Dr. Yeo (Charlie), and he reviewed with me the specifics of the surgery itself and my postoperative recovery regimen. He also had me sign a surgical consent form which had plainly written on it what the surgery was, why is was being done, and what the risks were. I signed it, trying to keep my cool and not cry as my pen marked the paper with my signature.

I had planned to ask him some questions about exactly what my incision would look like, but got too nervous to ask. It was probably just as well. There was no sense in dwelling on this subject longer than absolutely necessary. He had previously discussed with me the option of having reconstructive surgery done at the same time. I was a candidate for a tram-flap procedure, but not a candidate for implants. I had opted to not have that done and he had explained that by not choosing this additional procedure, I had not burned my bridges for opting to do it in the future. He even mentioned that some plastic surgeons prefer that patients wait six months and then have it done. The healing process is more optimal. I had very mixed feelings about this procedure and also a great concern about being under anesthesia for about eight to ten hours. I also didn't know if I wanted my abdominal flesh and vessels relocated onto my chest. It might have looked like a breast mound, but my brain would know that it wasn't. Anyway, I was glad that this option wasn't a "do it now or you lose your chance" kind of a procedure.

He explained that I would be going home about twenty-four hours after the operation, with two hemovacs. I was familiar with these devices, so no detailed explanation was needed.

Shortly before we had gone on vacation I had sent him a personal note thanking him for the time that he had spent with me on the phone and letting him know that I knew I was in good hands. I had also drawn a silly cartoon on the card for him to let him know I wasn't going to let this experience rob me of my sense of humor. He was very amused by my drawing and appreciated my card. That made me feel really good. I realized after I sent the card to him that maybe he would think I was some kind of a nut or something. But I was willing to run that risk to let him know more about me and my style of handling medical crises. I've drawn for you the same cartoon, or should I say riddle, that I drew for him. Here it is:

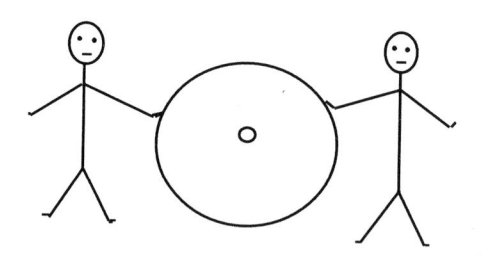

What is this a picture of?
Answer: It's two men walking "abreast."

Now is that funny or what? I sure thought so, and fortunately he did too.

I also realized that this physician was going to be and had already become a very important person in my life. He was the individual who was going to transform me from a cancer victim to a cancer survivor. It could have been done by someone else, but I had selected him to fulfill this role for me. He also would be one of the very few men in my life who would see me with only one breast—who would see me in the flesh, as they say. Only Charlie Yeo, my gynecologist, and my husband would see me this way. Other men in my life would have to play the guessing game of "which boob is it?" Charlie's attitude about women's breasts would be very influential to me. If he treated them like they were insignificant, then I would interpret that as possibly all of me as being insignificant. But if he made me feel that they were important but not as important as my life, then I would have found someone who thought as I did, as my husband did, and as my parents did. I was blessed . . . he did exactly that. With the utmost professionalism, he explained to me that he knew that losing my breast was a terrible thing. Having to be the surgeon to do this unpleasant deed was equally awful. But knowing that my life would go on as a result of it made it the right thing to do.

I had been in the presence of other surgeons before, when I was still working as a clinical nurse at the bedside, and had seen some who were caring and compassionate and some who were cold and seemingly uncaring of what a patient who was losing a breast was going through. I believe that surgeons have a very tough job when it comes to performing a mastectomy or any type of amputation. They have to be compassionate enough to have empathy for their patients while remaining objective and disconnected from the patient to perform an operation and keep their cool. Not all surgeons possess these qualities; that's why I chose so carefully. I had chosen well. I knew the first time I met with Charlie Yeo that he possessed these qualities. No doubt his mother was proud of him. I knew that my mother would love him too.

I remember one time I was in the operating room as a scrub nurse. The case I was to scrub in on was an above-the-knee amputation. The patient was in his mid-seventies and was a brittle diabetic. Despite numerous hospitalizations, debridements, and whirlpool baths, the man's leg continued to harbor a nasty infection that progressed into gas gangrene. The last option to really save this man's life and prevent him from getting sepsis and dying was to remove his leg. Because he had a bad heart, the anesthesiologist felt that he was at too great a risk to receive general anesthesia, so he was given a spinal anesthetic accompanied by hallucinogenic drugs. He would be awake but under the influence of powerful drugs during the operation; however, I was told that he would have absolutely no recall of it by that afternoon. When I came into the operating room that day, the patient was already on the table, prepped, and surgery was about to start. Usually in an operating room things are fairly quiet. The voices you hear are those of the surgeons asking for specific instruments to be passed to them. This surgery was different. The surgeon doing the case was an older, brassy, tough man who enjoyed giving nurses a hard time.

The procedure began. Instead of hearing only the voice of the surgeon, we heard the voice of the patient, in the literal sense. The patient started singing! As the doctor proceeded to cut the skin, tie off various blood vessels, and expose the bone, the patient sang and sang. He didn't seem to know that he was in an operating room at all. But I knew that he was and this entire experience completely unnerved me. Then the sawing began. The cutting of bone sounded and looked much like that of cutting a tree. Once it was cut through and the remaining flesh was severed, the leg was no longer attached to the man's body. It looked amazing to see this patient talking and singing and his leg being completely disconnected from his body.

The surgeon looked up at me and instructed me to pick up the limb and carry it to pathology down the hall. I was shaking when he made this request of me. I was amazed at myself that thus far I had passed all the instruments he had asked for without dropping or fumbling even one of them. But now this? One of the more senior nursing staff attempted to intercede for me and do this assignment, but he insisted that it was *my* job. I took in a deep breath and picked up the leg, holding it in my arms by supporting it under the knee and ankle. I held it away from my body. It felt warm. My stomach felt queasy. As I reached the door of the OR, the surgeon asked me to turn around so he could check something. He looked at the foot and said, "Yep, that's what I thought. Look, Miss Dierker, his toes are still wiggling." Well, I never got to look at those toes to verify what the man said to me. I heard those words and fell onto the floor like a tree being cut at its base. I fainted—leg and all, down I went.

When I came to, there were a lot of nurses standing over me and the leg was gone. One of the nurses said to me, "He shouldn't have done that to you. He was getting nervous himself and that was his way of releasing his tension. By refocusing everyone on you, he could forget for a moment that he had made this patient a crippled man. This gentleman has been a patient of his for years. It was very hard for him to have to take his leg off, but it had to be done."

I was given the opportunity to scrub in on a lot of surgeries over those next three months that I worked in the OR, but that was the only time I fainted in the operating room. I looked at that surgeon differently after that. I was still angry that he had pulled that trick on me. He said later, "Just lighten up, Miss Dierker; I was just pulling your leg. I mean making a joke. You take life too seriously." Well, I knew one thing: I didn't want to be in the operating room during a mastectomy. No sir. And whenever a mastectomy was booked, I always took a surgery scheduled in the other room during that block of time. Even though I knew I would not be in a situation again where the patient was euphorically awake, I didn't want to be asked to hold someone's breast and take it to the pathology department. I knew my stomach wouldn't be able to take it…nor would my heart. I feared that I would relate to it too much because of my friend, Miss Bertha. So I was spared that experience.

Being with these patients in the recovery room and out on the surgical nursing units tugged at my heart strings enough. Soon, though, there would be scrub nurses in the OR with me and I would be the patient. I felt bad for them and hadn't even met them yet.

I went to see Marla the day before my surgery. She gave me a gift. It was a lovely compact of pressed powder with a mirror. She told me that she was giving it to me so I could see myself after surgery and see what a breast cancer survivor's face looked like. She also told me that whenever she worried about her teenage daughters, she pictured them being in protective bubbles of light. Inside these bubbles, no harm could come to them and they would remain safe no matter what bad things were around them. She wanted me to picture myself in such a special bubble of light that night and when I went into surgery the following morning. She gave me her private phone number and asked that Al call her as soon as I was out of surgery and back in my room, fully recovered from anesthesia.

I picked up a videotape that Earl Steinberg, a key player also in my adjustment and recovery, had gotten from a friend of his. The tape was made by a breast surgeon at a major medical center in Boston. Still in its draft stages, it was a video designed to show women who have been diagnosed with breast cancer what the surgical scars look like. Its focus was on a comparison of lumpectomy surgery (also referred to as breast-sparing surgery) with mastectomy surgery. It also showed photos of what reconstructive surgery results looked like. The tape included interviews of women who had each type of surgery done and their feelings about the surgical options that they had chosen. Earl thought that perhaps this tape would be of use to me. He, like I, felt that information equaled power and control. He didn't know how best to help me from a medical perspective because this field of medicine was not his own. He wanted to do whatever was in his power to provide me resources to help me get through this experience. I was very touched by his sincerity and compassion. Up until then we had been primarily working colleagues. This experience moved us to a higher plateau. I was thankful for his friendship. Unfortunately, I lacked the nerve to watch the video prior to my own surgery. I thought, "What if I hear somebody say that the absolutely best way to have this cancer removed was to have a lumpectomy? Could I possibly be influenced by a voice of an unknown person?

What if someone on this tape said that women who don't have reconstruction done right away have suicidal tendencies? Would I believe such hogwash? Well, I had no idea what was on that tape. Though I believed it was probably a valuable reference for me, I elected not to watch it. I had made my decisions based on what I felt was the best medical advice that I could possibly receive. I decided that I would watch it after I was home and recovering from my surgery.

Al took me to Hunt Valley Mall that night, hoping to tire me out by walking around and touring through the stores. We were going to go to the movies, but that seemed like a waste of money. My mind would not have been on the show. We ran into two different people we knew and hadn't seen for a long time. These weren't really friends, but acquaintances. Each of these people asked how we were and we responded with the patent answer of "fine" and left it at that. We left the mall around closing time and drove home. My anxiety was building. I wondered if there was something that I should do before going to bed. Should there be some special ceremony to tell my breast good-bye? Should I take a picture? I decided that the answer was no. There was nothing to be done.

Dr. Beattie called me that night around ten o'clock. He had told me that he would. I wanted to talk with him and hear him say one more time that the anesthesia would be no problem. He did. He was wonderful. He asked me to try to get a good night's sleep so that I would be ready for him in the morning. I told him that I would try.

After I hung up with him, I turned on a cassette tape of some songs that my girlfriend, Wanda, and I had sung on my karaoke machine a few weeks before this experience started. It sounded good to hear us singing and even better to hear us laughing together. I wanted to hear us laughing again, after tomorrow was behind me. I thought once again how we take life for granted—how all of us all too often don't realize just how precious each happy moment is. Then Al and I went to bed.

It was eleven o'clock. The house was quiet. Laura was staying with my mother-in-law for the night. We had received many phone calls that day to wish me well and offer prayers for me. Everything that could be done had been done to make the next day go well. The minute hand on the clock moved slowly that night. I was up and down, walking around twice during the night. When I returned to bed the second time, I was thinking about Grandmother Dierker, my father's mother. She had died several years before and I still missed her.

As I drifted off to sleep, I felt someone rubbing my leg. I sat up in bed, but saw that no one was there. No one who I could see, anyway. I believe that my grandmother was there in the bedroom that night, letting me know I'd be okay.

Eventually the alarm clock went off at 4:45 A.M. I arose, took a shower, and got dressed. The house was extremely quiet. Neither Al nor I talked at all. We just offered silent gestures of hugs as we passed each other in the hall. I decided to wear comfortable clothes, so I dressed myself in my favorite blue shirt and a pair of shorts—certainly not the usual attire I wore to the work, but this day I wasn't going to the hospital as an employee. I was going as a patient.

We arrived at the hospital around 5:45 A.M. and I was due to report to the presurgical area at six. Al dropped me off at the door so that I could quickly use the bathroom. My stomach was grumbling and I knew that I would have the green-apple quick steps before I got up to the same-day surgery area. As I entered the hospital at that ungodly hour, I spotted someone whom I was very pleased to see. It was our hospital chaplain, Clyde Shallenberger. He inquired what I was doing here at this very early hour and why I was dressed funny. I took his hands and told him of my situation. He hugged me and said that he'd be by to see me after surgery and he'd pray for me (or, as he sometimes says it, "talk with his boss") while I was in the OR. I felt very much at peace, having run into him like that. I still have absolutely know idea what Clyde was doing there at that hour. I was certainly glad to see him, though. Perhaps the hour wasn't as ungodly as I had thought . . .

Al joined me just a few minutes later and we held hands as we took the elevator up to the fifth floor. There were about six families waiting outside of the pre-op area, waiting for the doors to be unlocked. Soon a nurse came and let us all go inside. One by one the receptionist called our names, and one by one each patient was identified from the group that he or she was seated with. Soon my name was called and I was given forms to fill out. As I completed them, my eyes kept drifting up; I watched two parents sitting with their small child. The child was about three and was mentally retarded. These two parents had the patience of a saint. The child was apparently the patient and therefore couldn't have anything to eat or drink. The little boy kept pointing to his mouth and crying. His mother picked him up and told him that he wasn't allowed to have anything and that she was sorry. He cried. Then she pulled out some toys from a large bag she had brought with her. One of the toys was a music box. She wound it up and gave it to him. He instantly stopped crying and held the box right up against his ear. He sat there on the floor and rocked himself to the music.

I looked at this family and realized how truly blessed I was. My child was normal. My family was healthy. And after this ordeal I too would be a well person, I hoped.

After a few moments went by, my name was called and I was escorted into an exam room. Al was allowed to come with me. There I was asked to remove my clothes and put on a hospital gown, hat, and booties. "We'll be wheeling you into the operating room from here, Mrs. Shockney, so you'll need to say good-bye to your husband now." Al leaned down and kissed me twice. "I love you. I'll see you soon." Tears began to flow down my cheeks. I prayed to God not to let me make a fool of myself when I reached the operating room. I had a terrible fear that I would turn into a screaming bantam chicken, pleading with the doctor not to proceed with the operation.

In a moment I was at the door of the operating room. I could hear the scrub nurses talking and the sounds of the equipment and stainless steel portable carts that hold instruments being wheeled into place. I was glad that my contact lenses were out of my eyes so the room looked unfocused. I didn't want to see any scalpels or other instruments. I was asked to stand and position myself onto the operating room table. My heart was racing.

Dr. Beattie came in and looked down at me. "Well, Lillie, how much sleep did you get for me last night?" I told him that I had the same amount that I had when I was in hard labor with my daughter at the time of her birth. He patted my hand. I got a grip on him and couldn't let go. He reassured me that all would go well. A resident was with him and he introduced him to me. His eyes were kind. He had the assignment of putting the IV in my hand.

Dr. Beattie then told me that he'd be giving me a drug called madazalam to make me feel good and that I'd forget my troubles within a few seconds of it being injected through my IV. As he injected the medicine, it burned. He tried to lighten my emotional load by telling me that this medicine would make me tell all of my secrets. It was an affective distraction too. I was suddenly no longer focused on my breast and instead worried that I might tell stories out of school. Then I closed my eyes and heard my mother singing in my head. She was singing a song that I used to enjoy hearing her sing at churches. It was called, "He Gazed Up and Smiled On Me." It was about a person meeting Christ along the side of the road. I felt perfectly calm now. I was here for a good reason, not a bad one. I was here to be transformed from a breast cancer victim to a breast cancer survivor. This is what I wanted. And with that I was asleep.

Chapter 12

The next voice that I heard was that of Dr. Beattie telling me that I was in the recovery room and that my surgery was over. I had trouble opening my eyes but could hear his voice plainly. I remember asking him if I had told any Hopkins' secrets and he reassured me that I hadn't. I believed him, but not completely. For all I knew, the surgical team had set up a microphone near my head to be guaranteed that any politically hot secrets that I might have known could be electronically recorded. I definitely wanted to be sure to get the next publication of the Hopkins Hotline to make sure that there wasn't a one-page spread dedicated to me entitled, "Director of QA tells all while under the influence of drugs."

I wanted to move my hands up to my chest but lacked the strength initially to do so. Finally I was able to slide both of my hands up to my chest. I placed one hand over each breast area. I felt nothing on either side! Just flatness. Flat as a pancake. I called out for a nurse to come. Any nurse. A young woman dressed in scrubs hastened over to me. "Are you in pain, Mrs. Shockney?" I told her no. I wanted to know what had been done to me. I couldn't feel either breast. What had happened? Had someone made a mistake and taken off the wrong one and then, in discovering this error, removed the one that we knew did have cancer in it? Or did the doctor get more information from the pathology department that made him biopsy the right breast and subsequently discovered that it too was cancerous? No, none of these things were true. She explained that my left breast was gone and that I had on a very tight binder that compressed the dressings tightly to prevent swelling. The binder went all the way around me so this was the reason that my right breast felt like it wasn't there either. What a relief! But as I concentrated in my mind to feel the sensation of my right breast (the remaining one) I realized that I still felt like my left breast was there too.

I asked the question again of the recovery room nurse. "Tell me just what exactly was done. Did Charlie do the mastectomy as planned?" She answered yes again. She then checked the hemovacs. I could see each of the drainage containers when she held them up to look at the amount of bloody fluid in them.

I looked around the room as best as I could, still woozy from the effects of the anesthesia. There were many stretchers with patients on them and lots of moaning sounds could be heard. My mind drifted back to my nursing experiences with recovery room patients...their confusion as to where they were...their grimaced looks of pain when they awakened.

Then I heard a woman moaning and yelling out beside me on the stretcher to my left. "Is it gone? Oh no, it is. It is. God help me." A nurse came over to her and took her hand. The patient didn't speak anymore, she just cried. The nurse didn't speak either. She just held the patient's hand and stroked her forehead. The woman soon drifted back to sleep. I then called the nurse over to me. "Is she okay? She sounded so upset." The nurse responded and her words came as no surprise to me. It was what I had surmised. I was laying beside a newly enlisted club member like myself. She, too, had had a mastectomy. The left side was gone, just like mine.

I wanted to turn over and look at her but my lack of strength prevented me from doing so. Soon she was taken away, taken out to the nursing unit where she would complete her recovery.

Complete her recovery...that really wasn't so, though. Neither of us was going to complete our recovery here at the hospital. Soon, we would be well enough to go home, but the majority of our recovery would take place far from these walls. I wanted to start working on those steps to recovery as soon as possible, too. My transformation was complete and it was time to focus my attention on getting well and getting on with my life. I never got to meet that other patient who had lain next to me. I hope that she did well and has been blessed with the necessary support systems it takes to get through those post-surgical steps to recovery.

My husband was allowed to come into the recovery room and be with me. I was told later that I had been calling out for him. I don't remember doing this, but often patients do things in the recovery room that they erase from their mind instantaneously. He was all smiles, with only a few hives on his face.

When Al is under stress, he gets hives. He looks like someone took red lifesavers and stuck them all over his face, so it's easy to see how high his stress level is by the number of red lifesavers I can count on his face. I remember when we bought our house and went to settlement. He had about fourteen or fifteen hives on his face. He was truly a lumpy bumpy mess. He had only a few until he saw how much money that we would truly be paying for our home by the time it was paid off thirty years from the date of settlement. By the time that he read the numbers and signed his name, the hives were all over his face and neck. Looking at him at the foot of my stretcher with all those lumps and bumps on his face made me worry that he knew something about how the surgery went that I didn't know. He reassured me that everything went fine and Dr. Yeo had spoken to him and to my parents and gave them a good report on me. The hives were from worrying that I'd have trouble with anesthesia, but he had been reassured by Dr. Beattie that all was well with that too. He looked very happy and just couldn't stop smiling at me and telling me that he loved me. Various nurses came over to him and told him that I was doing well. He'd just beam all the more.

Patients say very funny things sometimes. This time I was the one being funny rather than being the nurse that got to hear the funny things being said. Al told me that I kept telling everyone in the recovery room that I felt like something was standing on the left side of my chest. Upon inquiry, I further explained to those within hearing distance that an elephant was standing on my chest. When Al asked me about the elephant, I assured him that it was a little elephant, just a baby, and that it was okay for it to be there. Who knows, maybe I thought that I was Dumbo's mother.

I was eventually stable enough to be moved to my room out on the nursing unit. Al left me to make arrangements for the phone to be connected in my room and such. As I traveled down the hallway, my stomach felt queasy and I was relieved finally to be in a bed where I could position the head of my bed a little higher. Soon Al returned. Right behind him were my parents. Dad stood at the side of my bed. I said hello as if greeting people for some other sort of gathering. Dad was tearful. Mom looked relieved but very tired. Her five weeks of worrying was plainly visible on her face.

Dad didn't want to stay, but I insisted that they not rush off so quickly. I think he was afraid that he would get too emotional and not project the image of a tough guy. But he had been a tough guy in my book. A tough guy to me is someone who is strong when the going gets tough, and the going had gotten pretty tough for all of us. Mom and Dad kissed me. Each told me that they loved me. Mom said she'd see me tomorrow when Al brought me home. I wondered what had been racing through their minds after all these weeks of anguish and torture. Being parents is truly a lifetime job that requires you to be on call twenty-four hours a day. Surely they would both get good check marks in God's giant book for enduring this experience.

Right before Mom and Dad left, Al pulled out of his pocket a note that Laura had given to him. She had requested that it be given to me as soon as I was back in my room. It was all sealed up in an envelope; obviously it contained highly confidential material and was for selective viewing. I had Al open the envelope for me then I took the paper out and read it out loud. It was a poem. It was dated July 9, 1992, so I knew that she had written it five days before this day.

Appearance

Nobody's perfect;
Just look at me
But if you really think about it
Who wants to be?

Beauty and glamour
Are nice to get
But it's what's inside that counts;
You must never forget.

I hope you understand
What I've been trying to say

I hope you get well soon
And I love you more and more each day.

>Love,
>Laura

When your child who is all of twelve years of age writes something that is that philosophically marvelous, it's hard to have a dry eye in the room. As you can imagine, there were no dry eyes in my hospital room that afternoon. I thought it was wonderful that someone so young could be so wise. Children usually adjust well to crisis situations; they are so resilient. I wonder at what age we lose this wonderful way of viewing the world. I once again hoped and prayed that her analytical approach to dealing with this family crisis would never be tested out on her when she became an adult herself. I prayed, "Oh please, God, don't let this ever happen to my baby. She is too special to have to be confronted with such an unpleasant and evil thing as breast cancer."

I glanced up at my mother's face and understood, at least a little bit, just how devastating this experience must have been for her, and still was for her. She was aging with worry right before my eyes. As a matter of fact, a few nights before my surgery, my grandmother called me to talk for a while. She was worrying about my mother and how much older she appeared to have become in only a matter of weeks. She said, "She is worrying so. I know that you are going to be all right. She needs to sleep and worry less. I think that the wrinkles in her face are so bad now that Oil of Olay isn't even going to help." Just think of it—four generations of women, each one worrying about her daughter. It was amazing to think about it and even more amazing to be experiencing it. My folks left a few minutes later. I hoped that that night they would each worry a little bit less.

I soon started having visitors. First Diane, Scott, and Marge came by. They all looked relieved to see me and glad that my surgery was over. They didn't stay long so as not to exhaust me. I appreciated their consideration. They also ran interference for me to prevent an entourage of people from coming to my door. Though everyone meant well, having continuous visitation was not in my best interest at that time. They knew that and encouraged others to recognize this as well. They carried back status reports to my staff and other hospital employees who were anxious to know how things had gone.

Earl came by for a visit that evening. He was such a dear man. I knew that he had an unbearable schedule and, despite it, came by before he went home to see how I was doing. Tim also came by. So did Clyde. I told Clyde that his boss had done a good job and obviously had responded to the many requests (prayers) that had been submitted to him by various people on my behalf. He smiled and held my hand for a moment, then departed.

My stomach started misbehaving, and before long I was throwing up. I threw up about every ten to fifteen minutes from four until half past eight. Al patiently held the emesis basin as I'd give yet another heave. Eventually the antinausea medicine took effect and my stomach quieted down. I was offered pain medicine several times but did not feel the need to take it. Usually pain killers upset my stomach and I had done all of the throwing up I intended to do.

Al left around dark that night. I didn't want him to go, but he had to pick up Laura from his mother's and I knew that she needed time with him too. He had called everyone on our list of contacts to let them know that I was out of surgery and doing reasonably well. He was definitely operating off of nervous energy that day. He kissed me often and held my hand. It was a special night for us to share together.

A resident came in to see me from the surgical team shortly after Al left. He checked my bandages, which required him to unfasten my binder. I held my breath when he did this maneuver. I was afraid of feeling pain, but even more frightened that my eyes would be tempted to glance downward and look at the surgical site. It was no trouble resisting this temptation, though. He told me that he had been in the operating room with me that day. Though I had believed Dr. Beattie when he told me that I hadn't told any stories out of school, I was curious if I had said anything after I was drugged. He told me that I had made one request before I was completely under. That request was to be "reassembled" in the event that something went wrong and I didn't wake up. I must have been really frightened; I must have thought that I was like the character Number Five in the movie, *Short Circuit*.

For those of you who haven't seen this movie, Number Five was a computerized robot that had artificial intelligence. At least the scientists who created him thought that it was artificial. Later they discovered that he had somehow taken on human qualities and he could think on his own and feel emotion. In part of the movie there were strategic plans being made to capture him and disassemble him. When Number Five overheard the scientists discussing their plans, he said, "Disassemble? NO disassemble!" I found it curious that I would make such a last request. I guess my subconscious didn't want to give up my breast if it wasn't absolutely necessary. And if I were to die there on the operating table, there certainly would be no particularly good reason why it shouldn't be reattached and buried with me.

I recall telling a girlfriend of mine that if I opted to have reconstruction done and died on the operating table from an anesthesia complication, I would want to be laid out in my casket nude from the waist up. I'd want everyone to see just what I had died for. Heck, such a death would seem completely senseless to me if friends didn't get to see what I was willing to sacrifice my life for. They could say, "Well, would you look at the bodacious tah tahs on Lillie. She wasn't really ever happy with having to settle for only having one left. Well, she didn't get to see the new one but she sure would have been pleased with it."

At approximately 9:30 P.M., a strange woman entered my room. She was carrying a large plastic bag and her purse. She came over and introduced herself. She was a Reach to Recovery volunteer. I was surprised to see her there so late, but welcomed the opportunity to visit with her. She sat at my bedside and spoke very softly. As she spoke, she slowly removed objects from her plastic bag.

First she pulled out a small pink cotton rectangular pillow and offered to place it under my left elbow. She said that these pillows were made by volunteers and were designed to provide a little extra support for my affected arm. Next she took out some reading material that contained information about places to buy prosthesis, mastectomy bras, wigs for patients who go through chemotherapy, and a list of support groups in the immediate area. She asked me about my experience with breast cancer thus far—about how was I diagnosed, if I planned on reconstruction, whether the doctor anticipated chemotherapy, and so on. Next she took out a bra that appeared to be something like a sports bra but much stretchier and softer. She explained that when the doctor said

I could come out of my binder and have the hemovacs removed, I would be able to wear this as a bra until I was ready to be fitted for a breast prosthesis. Usually, most surgeons prefer that the patient be at least six to seven weeks post-op before they go for a fitting. This way the fitting can be done correctly and without interference of chest and arm edema. She showed me how to make a temporary prosthesis from cotton batting that she had brought along with her and she shaped a breast prosthesis for me while she was there and showed me how to put it in and out of the pocket of the mastectomy bra that she had given me. I wore a 42D bra and felt very strange seeing this mastectomy bra with a large wad of cotton in it. It really started to hit me that my breast was really gone. Tears began to silently stream down my face.

The Reach to Recovery volunteer stayed with me for about an hour and a half. I appreciated her visit very much. I had the opportunity to talk face to face with another club member about my concerns and worries.

Once the volunteer left, the room was, for the first time all day, quiet and free of visitors. I felt a little uncomfortable being alone. I didn't want to be in there without anyone. I think I was afraid that, if left alone, I'd have too much time to reflect about the events of the day. My mind was overwhelmed as it was. Thank heavens the door to my room opened and Jean came in. Jean was the breast cancer nurse specialist. She was working very late that day and stopped by to see how I was doing. She checked my dressings and told me that Dr. Yeo would be there in the morning to review with me his discharge instructions and describe how he wanted me to record my hemovac drainage. I told her that Al would be in early in the morning, but the person who would be helping me with the dressings would be my mother. I would be able to show her what needed to be done. I told her that I wasn't ready for Al to look at my incision yet and she said that this was okay. Shortly thereafter she left my room. I was impressed that she had taken the time to come by to see me, particularly at that late hour.

It was now approaching eleven, the time for change of shift. Myck, a very attractive Asian nurse, poked her head in to see me one last time before she went out for the evening shift report. She checked the amount of fluid left in my IV bag. Just as she prepared to leave, I started to cry. I don't know exactly what I was crying about. There were so many reasons to cry that I'm not even sure I singled out any particular one to initiate the flood that rolled down my face. Despite the fact that the evening shift report was due and more patients' IVs needed to be checked and other duties needed to be attended to, Myck did what I used to pride myself in doing when I used to work at the bedside as a clinical nurse. She recognized that her patients' emotional needs were her priority. She sat down on my bed and took my hand. She just sat. No words, no glancing at her watch that her shift was over. She waited for me to speak. I think she would have waited with me all night had I not spoken and expressed what was on my mind. I said, "I've taken care of many patients in my life…many patients who have had done what has been done to me. I've sat on the bed with these patients as you are with me and held their hands and cried with them. I never once imagined that someday someone would be sitting in a white uniform with me." Tears ran down Myck's face, too. She didn't speak. We embraced and I reassured her that I would be all right and asked that she finish her rounds and give report. She stood by my bed for a moment longer, squeezed my hand, and told me that she wished me well. She then departed.

That was one of the longest nights of my life. I slept very little, it seemed. Each time I would awaken, I would get myself reoriented as to where I was and why I was there. My recovery from this ordeal would definitely require more than a bathtubful of Calgon bubbles. Oh, Calgon, take me away . . .

Chapter 13

I watched the sun as it rose through my window. The nursing unit was just starting to have some activity. I could hear the nursing staff talking in the hall and the sound of stretcher wheels as the night shift did their final activities of the early morning, prepping the patients who were going to surgery that morning. Soon my door swung open and Al walked through. What a welcome sight he was. He kissed me and asked me how my night had been. Just as he sat down beside me, the day-shift nurse came in and removed the IV from my hand. She told us that the surgical team would soon be in and would change my bandages before I went home. She also said that she would be back in shortly after breakfast to show Al how to empty my hemovac drainage bags.

"I don't want you in the room when the surgeons come in to change my dressings. Your job will be to manage the hemovacs. Mom and I will worry with the bandages. Deal?" I said very firmly. Al nodded in agreement and I felt relieved.

Since I had not been very successful in keeping a lot of food down from the anesthesia, I only had liquids for breakfast, but they slid down easily, thank goodness. Just as I finished, the nurse came back in and started her discharge instructions regarding the drains. They had to be emptied four times a day and the amount of drainage measured and recorded on a paper that she gave us. She showed Al how to empty the drain labeled #1 and then he emptied the #2 drain under her supervision. He did fine—nervous, but fine. The nurse had just left the room when the door swung back open to reveal Charlie Yeo.

He was chipper and dressed in scrubs and his long white coat. He swiftly walked over to me and before I could answer his question of how my night had been, he had maneuvered himself into a sitting position beside me on the bed and unfastened my binder. I was petrified. It happened so fast, it seemed. Then, before I could prepare for my defense, he asked Al to come over and help him change my dressings. My heart was racing and my palms were sweating. I was unable to speak. I wanted to yell out, "Hey. Wait just a cotton pickin' minute. This isn't the deal. I don't want my husband to see my incision yet!" But I was unable to get my lips to move. As Charlie removed all of the bandages, I could feel the coolness of the air on my chest. My eyes were fixed on Al's face. I was watching his every move, every blink, waiting to see a look of disgust, a look of rejection. I only saw a look of seriousness. He wanted to make sure that the way he was putting the new bandages on the wound met with the physician's approval. I don't think I could have felt worse if a team of doctors had come into my room, stood me on my head naked, spread my legs, and used a protoscope to look up my rear end while video taping the entire procedure onto a fifty-inch TV screen that was set up in the main corridor of the hospital for all to see. It was awful. But when it was over, Al looked up at me and said, "It looks fine. We're going to be fine." I knew then that Charlie had perhaps done one of the best things that he could have ever done for me, for us.

By showing Al how he wanted the dressings changed each day, he had also shown me that we were going to be okay. My scar was not going to be a barrier to our maintenance of a good relationship and marriage. I still don't know if Charlie does this with all the husbands or if he sizes up the situation and makes that judgment call as the circumstances allow him. He is a clever man. For all I know, they both planned the whole thing. It doesn't matter now. It's in the past. But it's a moment I will always remember. (I'm still annoyed that I didn't get to see Al without his teeth, though. I was cheated out of that Kodak moment.)

Scott and Diane came up to the room just as we were preparing to leave. Their timing was perfect. This gave Al the opportunity to go down alone and get the car and bring it to the front entrance while these two special friends escorted me down in the wheelchair. I wore my shorts that I had worn to the hospital and a large (better described as jumbo, size forty-eight) button-up shirt that I had purchased especially for this day. Because my hair gets very oily at night I wore a hat too and I wore my glasses. Even if an employee who knew me well were to see me, I doubt he would have recognized me. As a matter of fact, quite a few people who I knew were in the hallway and walked right on by me. I was very relieved about that. Soon I was out to the car and tucked safely into the front seat for the ride home. Scott, Diane, and I must have looked like we were saying good-bye for a decade. No one's eyes were dry.

Once we reached home Mom came out to help us get all of our gear into the house. She still looked as if she had gotten little sleep and it was clear that her migraine headaches had persisted. I felt awkward walking around with the drainage hoses safety-pinned to my shirt. I had a constant fear that the pin would pop and the drain would rip right out of my chest cavity. Even though I knew they were sutured in, I worried. I told people that the hemovacs felt like hand grenades; if I were to make the wrong move, then *POW!*

Laura was glad to see me. She gave me a kiss. Because of her weak stomach, she didn't ever stay in the room very long. "See, you said that you would look different, but you don't to me. Other than you wearing your glasses instead of your contact lenses, you look just the same," she said. I told her that I looked different under my clothes. She was unimpressed. She simply replied by telling me that no one could see under there, "so it doesn't count."

Mom helped me change into a nightgown. I had purchased three gowns. They were one size fits all. These gowns were smart investments for me. They had a very large head opening and scooped-out neckline, and they were very full and flowing. There was ample room for me and my surgical army weapons.

We were only home about twenty minutes when the doorbell rang. It was a local florist bringing me a gorgeous bouquet of flowers. The doorbell rang a lot that week. Between flowers and balloons, I received over twenty get-well wishes. I also received during that week other special treasures like a stuffed cow, a whimsical cow pin, cow eggs, stuffed bunnies, baskets, fragranced soap, books, and other lovely gifts—each from someone very special to me. (See Chapter 20 for a list of recommended gifts for a club member that you might know.)

Being surrounded by so many lovely bouquets of flowers and other well-wishing memorabilia was very uplifting to my spirits. The messages on the gift cards were also special and I have retained every one. I also took pictures of the floral arrangements. Usually to receive so many exquisite bouquets you have to be dead; how fortunate I was to receive and enjoy them.

My first night home was a restless one. Al decided that I should have the bed to myself so he slept downstairs on the sofa. Mom was in Laura's room. I placed two pillows under my head and one between my knees. To support my left arm, my surgical side, I used one more pillow. I also kept my little pink pillow, made by the Reach to Recovery volunteers. It made me feel close to club members even though there were none around.

The next morning Al and Mom helped me get up and moving. I had now gone two and one half days without washing my hair and it really distressed me. I wasn't able to do anything about it, though.

Get-well cards started coming in. I read each one with great care. I saved them all. Before two weeks would pass, there would be over two hundred cards delivered to our mailbox. I was amazed.

The phone rang often, of course. Mom and Al got things down to a science when it came to helping me get around in the house, fixing meals, answering phones, and opening mail. Cards are very special to me. I love sending cards. For that matter, I love reading cards. I can stand in a card store for several hours and laugh my head off reading humorous cards. I'm the one you see in the stores who becomes so hysterical with laughter that I feel compelled to share the humorous moment, so I will walk up to a total stranger and show her the card that I just read. Sometimes people read it and also laugh; other times they just stare at me and walk away. Oh well, their loss. Below are some of the lines from a few of the cards that I received. Unfortunately, I can't show you the accompanying picture on the front of each card, but trust me, it was perfect for the verse.

Some favorite lines from my get well cards are:

Remember, when you're feeling so low you have to reach up to touch bottom...whose bottom it is can make a big difference!

I know things look tough right now. But hang in there. Otherwise, I'll be forced to call you and sing "High Hopes" really loud and off key.

Some days it's tougher to hang in there than others. Like the days you wear a really old bra with worn elastic.

Sometimes a friendly little smile can make your day . . . but usually it takes money or sex.

Wouldn't it be nice if our lives were like VCRs . . . and we could "fast forward" through the crummy times?

Relax. Things could be worse. You could be stuck in a hot elevator with a bunch of gross guys who went to an all-you-can-eat burrito buffet for lunch.

Aw, c'mon! Cuddly-Wuddly Bear wants you to cheer up! Kinda makes you wanna squeeze Cuddly-Wuddly Bear's little neck until his itsy-witsy button eyes pop off, doesn't it?

Remember: You're not fully dressed without a smile . . . oh, and underpants.

It's awfully hard to feel bad when you open a card that says something that tickles your funny bone just right. I also received a lot of lovely inspirational cards—cards that focused on the value of friendship, family, and religion. All of these cards are kept in a wooden basket that Diane brought me as a gift. I still look through them periodically and read the messages written to me by so many dear friends.

All in all, we were managing fairly well in the Shockney household. Don't get me wrong, there were still a lot of tears shed, but there was also a lot of laughter. One of the funniest moments came on my third day home. I couldn't stand my hair being glued to my scalp anymore and decided that it was time for a shampoo. I couldn't get in the shower, though, because of my bandages, and I couldn't lean over the sink either. It was a dilemma, but one I was determined to solve. Improvisation was the name of the game. While Al was outside getting the newspaper and Mom was in Laura's room getting dressed, I grabbed a hefty trash bag from the kitchen and proceeded to cut a whole in it for my head. When Al and Mom next saw me I was shrouded up in a dark green hefty bag with just my head sticking out. "Come! We're all going to wash my hair!" Into the shower we all went. We put a folding chair in the shower stall and Al held the shower head in his hands. I bent over as far as I could and mom kept towels around my neck in case of leakage around the opening in the bag. We laughed a lot that morning. Al said to me, "Well, don't you look like a prize right now . . . wrapped up in a hefty bag like an escaped lunatic." I told him that I was a prize—a booby prize. It was at that moment that I renamed my hemovac drainage bags booby traps! I felt great after my hair was washed. I looked better too. And each morning until I gained shower privileges I got my hair washed using the hefty bag system. I looked like a modern art version of a bag lady.

On Friday, just four days after my mastectomy was done, the drainage had dramatically subsided. I had my first appointment with Charlie that morning for him to check my hemovacs and decide if they could be removed. I wanted these booby traps gone but was afraid of what it would feel like having them yanked out. Charlie was there to see me within five minutes of my arrival. He took me in the exam room by myself and requested that my family wait in the reception area. He unveiled the incision and read the notes that we had meticulously kept of the drainage amounts from each container. He decided that the drainage was decreased enough that it was okay to pull both drains. Usually he kept in one of the drains for seven days, but he would be going out of town and felt that my risk of developing a seroma (a pocket of fluid that can form along the incision or in the axillary area) was minimal and worth chancing it. He had me lie on the exam table and asked me to hold onto the railings of the table while he pulled the first hose out.

He said, "Now, keep your hands on the side rails and don't move them. I'm afraid that if you move them, you'll locate them up to my throat." With that he pulled the first hose. It only took a second. My chest vibrated as he removed a hose that was equal in length to a garden snake. Then he pulled the second one. Finally I was free of these crazy contraptions and felt one step closer to recovery.

He was pleased with my healing thus far. I told him that I had my father's skin and usually did heal well with just a fine line of a scar. He asked me how things were going and I told him okay. He asked if I had looked at the incision yet and I told him no. He didn't press the issue.

I also told him about my phantom-limb sensation and phantom limb pain. He seemed intrigued with this. I told him that, just the evening before, I had been sitting at the kitchen table for dinner when suddenly I felt like someone was gently biting my nipple. My nipple that was no longer there. I told him that it seemed so weird to me. I didn't know what to say to my family about it. My mother knew that something wasn't quite right with me by the expression on my face. I elected not to say anything but I felt embarrassed so I got up from the table and went into the bathroom until the feeling went away. He smiled at me and said, "I bet you didn't tell your mother." He was right!

My mother went home that afternoon. She had stayed through the worst of my recovery period and was ready to head back home to the farm where Dad had been fending for himself for the last four days. There was no doubt in my mind that he was eating a lot of sweets and treats while she was over helping to take care of me.

The following morning I decided that it was time for me to look at my incision. I had Al hold up a mirror while I unfastened the binder and peeled off the bandages. Despite the fact that I had cared for other patients who had had this same surgery done, I was shocked at the sight of the incision. I had pictured it in my mind many times, but seeing it for real was overwhelming; tears silently streamed down my face. Al reassured me that he thought it looked okay. I just kept shaking my head no and continued to look in the mirror. It was really gone. Even though it felt like it was still there, it wasn't. There was nothing there now but a long scar signifying that once there had been something there. I had to concentrate my mind on the reason as to why it wasn't there. The flesh that had been there had cancer in it, and, if left to its own volition, it would kill me. I had lost my breast in exchange for God sparing my life. I then realized that this was a very fair exchange, but one that would require more mental adjustment. In time it would be okay.

About ten days after my surgery, I was granted the privilege of removing the binder and keeping it off. No seromas had formed, which pleased me. I was finally able to wear the bra that the Reach to Recovery volunteer had brought me. I took it out of the bag and looked at it. I then felt the cotton batting that she had placed inside the left pocket of the bra cup. My girlish figure had been traded in for stuff and fluff. It certainly didn't feel like a breast, but it would have to serve as a substitute until the real artificial breast prosthesis was obtained. I added some more cotton batting and tried it on, then took it off again and tried to adjust the shape of the cotton in the cup of the bra to look something like a breast.

Before I put the bra back on, I glanced down at my feet. Good grief! I could see my feet! I had not been able to stand up straight and look down and see my feet since I had been fourteen years old. The left foot was in plain view; the right one was only in partial view due to the obstruction by my remaining right breast. I found this amazing.

Next I went into the bathroom and decided to clip my toenails. Suddenly what had been an awkward task in the past was simple because I could see my toes and reach for them without my boobs being in the way. Boy, do men have it easy. Then I returned to the bedroom and put on my soft stuff-and-fluff bra. I looked in the mirror. It wasn't a bad disguise, considering what it was made of. I put on a loose-fitting shirt. Al was quite impressed too. Yes, this would serve as an acceptable disguise until better provisions could be made. It was funny; I found myself forgetting, if only for a few seconds, that my breast was gone. I was on the road to recovery for sure now. Yes, there would be more bumps in the road ahead, but I felt thankful for the progress that I had made.

Chapter 14

I felt well enough to start taking short rides in the car with Al and Laura. We took trips to the store for ice cream, quick jaunts to the bank. I seemed to lack the energy for long outings. I also worried that people would bump into me and hurt my chest. There were times that I felt like making a sign and wearing it on my chest that said, "Danger. Standing too close to this object could be dangerous for your health." I thought that this would be an appropriate sign because I knew that if anyone bumped me and hurt my incision, I would deck the person for sure. Perhaps another sign would have been more self-explanatory: "This may appear to be a boob, but it isn't. Getting too close to it could jeopardize your personal safety."

I also worried that strangers could see that this was merely stuff and fluff and not a real breast. It didn't bounce at all. As a matter of fact, the bra on the left side had the tendency to ride up since no weight held it down. I did experiment with putting quarters in it to help give it a little weight but it rode up on my chest anyway. I felt that people were probably looking at me and wondering why one breast was two inches higher than the other one. I was constantly asking Al if my breasts were lined up all right. When you get right down to it, probably no one was looking at my chest at all, but you would not have been able to convince me of that at the time.

By my third week I felt anxious to start having work brought out to me from the hospital. Several of my employees would alternate making deliveries and picking up completed work on a daily basis. Though my energy level was still low, it made me feel good to feel productive and back in the working environment again. It also was good to have visits from my staff. Marge became a regular visitor and she, Diane, and Scott would leave some really funny notes for me that would keep me laughing when I felt like crying.

One afternoon, Al decided to take me out to the movies. This was to be my first venture out for more than a quick pit stop somewhere. The three of us went to see, *Death Becomes Her*. It was great! Black humor at it's best! Here were two young women about my age who would do anything to ensure that their bodies remained looking like those that belonged to a voluptuous twenty-one-year-old. They paid an extraordinary amount of money to receive a potion that guaranteed them a return to youth for eternity. Of course there was a catch to this marvelous miracle—they would live forever as well, and they had to be very careful with their bodies. When they hurt themselves, they would not heal in the usual way; to compensate they repaired themselves with things like crazy glue and lots of flesh tone #9 spray paint. It was really funny. These two ladies showed that vanity will kill you or make you wish you were dead in the end. Growing old gracefully is not too popular. Of course, now that I had walked by death's door myself, my own goal had been revised: I simply would be happy to grow old . . . grace would be nice but not required.

I had lots of visitors—Al's family and mutual friends. Jack, Al's older brother, came by daily on his way home from work. Each step of my progress he celebrated with us. Al and I had talked a lot about the possible reactions that some of our company might have. He was concerned that people would be lost for words and feel uncomfortable talking about my illness. He also worried that people would glance at my chest and this would upset me. I had thought this too and knew that it was perfectly natural for someone to drop their eyes to my chest. It was almost an impulsive reaction and I didn't find it offensive because I had expected it. I must admit, though, that I had more respect for those who didn't take a quick peek while I was looking at them. The stuff-and-fluff bra was a real confuser for some visitors, too. No one asked me which side was taken away. I'm sure that some had made bets about which side it was, though, and tried to figure it out. Between my loose-fitting shirts and cotton batting, it was hard to tell unless someone paid attention and was able to notice that suddenly things I had routinely done with my left arm I now did with my right.

Jack Murphy and his wife Linda came by to visit us one evening. This was truly one of my most enjoyable evenings. Jack and I have been close for years and his wife is as wonderful a person as he is. They brought me flowers and a gift of a huge beach towel with my name embroidered on it. "We want you to be getting ready for the beach as soon as you are able so that we can all spend some time in the sun on the sandy beach of Ocean City." They didn't ask me any questions about my health but instead waited for me to bring up the subject. We spent about two hours together, talking and laughing. Though I was very tired when they left that evening, it was a lovely night and one that I will remember. Jack had lost his brother to cancer not long before I was diagnosed and it was painstakingly clear that he didn't want to lose me. Al and I talked after they left that evening about how blessed we felt to have such dear friends.

Shirley stopped by quite often, too. She wouldn't stay very long so as not to tire me out, but always knew just what to say. I often would cry when she would come. Of course, one of Shirley's best features is letting friends cry on her shoulder and giving them comfort and complete acceptance. She, also being a nurse, knew surgically what I had been through. Shirley is a very large-busted woman and she was empathetic to the fact that part of my image was focused on my breasts.

Once, when she and I were taking a walk in the woods, we suddenly realized that we had unknowingly walked through a bed of ticks. They were literally everywhere—on our pants, on our shirts, arms, socks, shoes. We were furiously trying to remove as many as we could from each other. We then resorted to removing our shirts to get the ticks off that had gone into our clothing. Though we were only about twenty feet off the road, modesty was the last thing on our minds! We continued to remove ticks that were on our bras and in our bras. When we hastily returned to our cottage where we were staying, our husbands came up from the waterfront to see why we were back so soon. They each privately assisted us in removing any remaining ticks that were on our backs, behind our ears, and in our undergarments. Of course they found this most entertaining and felt very regretful that they had missed our strip act on the highway the hour before. From that day forward, both Al and Shirley's husband, Jim, would make jokes about performing tick checks. Obviously, it would be easier to check me for ticks now. There wouldn't be any ticks running around lost in my cleavage anymore. My surgery had included the invisible removal of my cleavage.

One evening after company had left and I was getting ready for bed, I came out of the bathroom with just my underpants on. Lying at my feet on her big cozy dog bed was Lady, our black labrador. Lady had an unpredictable habit of running away periodically. She would jump the fence in the afternoon and not return until the wee hours of the next morning. Lady is old and has no street sense, so we get very concerned when she does this. Actually, she is so old that it seems as if it is a miracle that she can even jump the fence. But she does, so we often spend the night worrying like the parents of a teenaged girl who is out in a car with a boy who has long hair and tattoos and who tells you, "Hey man, I'll get her home okay. Don't worry." The worrying begins the moment that the person is out of your sight and it doesn't cease until your daughter has arrived home and is inspected for damages and safely tucked away in bed. Then you can turn your worry glands off. Well, when Lady jumps the fence my worry glands become activated and don't turn off until she is back inside our home, lying on her bed all in one piece.

Now, I don't know exactly how much Lady understands when we talk to her but I know that she is fairly smart, so when she looked up at me and I said, "Do you see this scar? Well, this is what is going to happen to you if you ever jump that fence again and run away." I think she understood. The poor dog cowered down, put her tail between her legs and crawled out to the hallway where she slept most of the night.

I felt confident that I had surely cured her of the compulsion to jump the fence.

I had made an agreement with my surgeon, Charlie Yeo, to wait until his return from vacation to get my final pathology results from my surgery. Though it would have been preferable to have had the results as soon as possible, Charlie preferred to review the information with me personally rather than having one of his colleagues discuss it with me in his absence. So we made a pact that I would wait for his return and would not log onto the computer myself or ask someone else at work to give me a preview of the results. Though the waiting was hard, the fear of looking at the results myself again was overwhelming. I was sure that if I logged onto the computer, the Grim Reaper would appear and point his ugly finger at me. No, it was best for me to wait. I had an appointment with Charlie when I hit my three-week mark. It was his first day back to work and despite his very heavy schedule he gave me his undivided attention as always. He also gave me the kind of news that my family and I had been waiting for: my lymph nodes were clean. I was in stage one. What wonderful words to hear! Everyone was thrilled with the news. It was equal to, if not more exciting than, when we announced the birth of our child twelve years before. When I think about it we were really announcing a birth of a different nature. Perhaps it would be best to describe it as my rebirth. I was now officially a cancer survivor. We went home and called everyone to share the good news. When Jack, Al's brother, got word, he rapidly appeared with a half-bushel of steamed crab. This time there would be a happier ending for him, too. This time the person he knew so very well and who also shared the name Shockney, as his late wife did, would survive.

As the days progressed I felt stronger and more comfortable with my new body image. When I was four weeks post-op I decided that it was time for Laura to look at my incision. We had her sit in the middle of our bed with lots of space around her in case she fainted. I slowly took off my clothes until my incision was exposed. She stared at my incision. She studied it and studied it but said nothing. The silence was more than I could take, so I finally asked her what she thought about it. Her comments on seeing the results of her mother getting breast cancer were succinct but very powerful. She said, "I want to stay young." I realized how hard this must have been for her to have to deal with. It had only been a week before my surgery to have my breast removed that I had taken her to the department store to get her fitted for bras for herself. I asked her if she was worried that this would happen to her and she said, "No. Not right now, I'm not worried. I might get worried when I'm older, but I'm not worried right now."

I was worried though. How would I feel if I had passed this kind of cancer on to my child? Well, perhaps there will be a cure by the time she is my age. I realized at this particular time how important it was for her to see how I coped and adjusted. Perhaps if she could see that my life would go on and perhaps even in a better way than it was before, then she would somehow benefit from it, I thought. I knew that I would become active in the government and also with local groups who were diligently working hard to find cures for breast cancer as well as provide support for those who would become club members after me; she added to my inspiration to do these things.

I received phone calls from Earl, my physician friend at work, regularly. He called several times a week to see how I was doing. One day I was a little down and I said, "Well, Earl, I looked in the mirror and saw what I could go as for

Halloween this year. If I wear my birthday suit I'm sure to win first prize for the scariest costume." He was another friend who knew just what to say and when to say it so that I didn't stay down in the dumps very long. One evening when he called me he said that he had a favor to ask of me. Though it was only a couple of weeks since my surgery, he wondered if I would be willing to talk with a friend of his who had just been diagnosed with breast cancer that week. He thought that maybe I could be of some help to her. I was very flattered at his confidence in me. It was also very exciting to me. I was being given the opportunity to help a new club member—someone who had only just been drafted into the club. My response to his request was an overwhelming "YES!"

He had her call me the following day. She and I talked on the phone almost daily for about two weeks, which was up to the time of her surgery date. I also sent her funny cards in the mail and wrote down for her some suggestions of things to do before she had her surgery as well as things to do after her surgery. I mailed her small items in the cards that I sent her, like a one-time application of an antistress facial mask, a book mark with an inspirational phrase on it, a sachet for her lingerie drawer, and other feminine things that I hoped cheered her up. They did, too. She appreciated the gifts and cards and my words of wisdom about techniques to help her get through the days ahead. I realized that each step she took to cope with the diagnosis, to her transformation surgery, to getting on her road to recovery, also helped me down my own road to recovery. I realized that breast cancer survivors who were volunteers were not just giving; they were also getting a lot from the women whom they spent time with. I knew then that this new club member would be the first of many new club members whom I would spend time with and help along our very scary path as best as I could. It was a special privilege to help her and I looked forward to having opportunities to help others in the future.

Chapter 15

Al had been sleeping in a sleeping bag next to our bed for several weeks before he felt comfortable lying in bed with me. I was worried that he would bump my chest and he was worried about that too. I needed him close to me, though, so we had resorted to his sleeping on the floor. He must have felt like he was at summer camp or something. After about two to two and a half weeks or so we tested out having him resume his designated spot in the bed. I think the first night that he slept beside me neither one of us slept very well—each afraid that something would go wrong. He was experienced with having to be careful with me in bed. I have broken many bones in our fifteen years of marriage together and he has tried to lie beside me with casts on my legs and my arms, slings and immobilizers on my torso, and a variety of other contraptions that are not conducive to sleep. We were anxious to resume our normal sleeping routine, though, so we decided to give it a try. If ever there was a time that I wanted the man that I loved close to me, it was now. I needed that reassurance that I was loved and that the absence of my left breast didn't result in my being loved less.

We also talked about the best time to resume our sexual relationship. I realize that it was probably preferable just to let nature take its course but I had the distinct feeling that I was going to derail nature's plans unless things were carefully planned out. I wanted to have time to prepare myself, to think positive thoughts, to feel that the timing was right. It was almost like starting over for me. I looked at my husband as if he were a stranger of sorts and that I was also an unknown to him. We had planned to have an intimate encounter about three weeks after my surgery on a night that Laura was sleeping over at a friend's house. It was very late and I was extremely nervous. Al was equally nervous. We probably looked like two teenagers fumbling in the back seat of a car, scared. I was afraid of rejection; he was afraid of hurting me. He made every effort to be cautious of not leaning on my chest at all. I tried to focus on his face to see if I got any signals that my missing breast was a turn-off.

It was a tense night. I can't say that it was extremely pleasurable. It was okay. It would have been fine if I had been more trusting and believing of Al when he told me that my mastectomy didn't make any difference to him—that it didn't make me less of a woman to him. I needed proof, though, and felt that this night would be the real test. As I look back on it now, it was a miracle that he was able to perform at all, I think. If he looked the wrong way, or moved in a different manner, I questioned it. The first time was definitely the roughest, physically and emotionally.

As time went by and we relied on nature taking its course, we were able once again to experience the kind of closeness and intimacy that we had had before and could now enjoy again. Al would say to me, "When I press my chest up against yours now, our hearts can be closer to one another."

I often thought about other club members and wondered if they, too, had experienced the same kind of anxiety that my husband and I had in relation to resuming intimacy. I also thought about the patient who also had the phantom-limb sensation as I did now. As time went by and my incision became less tender, Al would gently touch it. Before too long we were also playing the new game of "In Search of the Missing Nipple." It is a fun game usually and certainly a great tension breaker on nights when I am feeling slightly self-conscious about my new appearance.

Laura began getting very quickly adjusted to my new body image too. She would come into the bathroom while I was taking a bubble bath and look at my incision. She even told me that she had gotten used to seeing me with only one breast and thought that I looked pretty good that way.

When I finally hit six weeks, I was eligible to be fitted for a breast prosthesis. Good-bye, stuff and fluff! I had made an appointment at a store called We Fit, which was only about twenty minutes from my home. It is recommended to take someone whom you are close to who will give you an honest critique of how the prosthesis looks on you when you go to be fitted. I decided to take my mother. Al was at first disappointed that I had not decided to take him, but I told him that I felt it was important to take a woman with me. I'd be in a room with other mastectomy patients and the store had recommended that I bring a woman whom I could trust to give me useful and accurate feedback. Well if you can't trust your mother then whom can you trust? Besides, I felt that this would be a positive experience for my mother too. She was still worried about me, wishing that none of this had happened to me, somehow wanting to be able to make me whole again. When I called and asked her if she would be willing to go with me, she said she would be honored to be there with me.

Mom and I arrived at the We Fit store at about ten in the morning. The shop was very busy that morning, with lots of women buying all kinds of undergarments. This particular store sells all kinds of lingerie, underpants, bras, girdles, etc., and they specialize in women who are hard to fit. I approached the counter and told the lady behind the desk that I was there for a prosthesis fitting. She ushered me to the back of the store where the fitting rooms were. Mom followed me.

When I got into the dressing area, the woman waiting on us introduced herself. She was an older woman and very soft-spoken. She asked me how many weeks ago I had had my surgery to confirm that I was at least six weeks post-op. She also asked me if my surgeon had approved my fitting and I handed her my prescription from his office. (The prescription simply says to fit me for a breast prosthesis. It doesn't limit you to a particular kind or anything. Surgeons are smart enough to leave this to the fitter and the patient.) The fitter then asked me to undress from the waist up, which I did. She looked at me with no look of surprise at all as I exposed my ten-inch incision that stretched across my chest from my breast bone to my armpit. She stared at my incision for a second or two, then said, "You look like a 42 C or D. I think that you'll take an Amoena, size nine." Size nine? What is she talking about? Am I buying Italian shoes or an artificial breast? With that, she stepped over to a huge closet that had French doors on it and proceeded to open it up. Inside there were hundreds of boxes. They looked like oversized shoe boxes. As I looked at them I read the writing on the side of them. Amoena, size nine left. Amoena, size seven, right. There were literally hundreds of prostheses in the closet—all shapes, all sizes, and a variety of brands. The fitter took down three boxes, sizes eight, nine, and ten, and brought them to my dressing room. She had me try on a mastectomy bra as well. She put the size nine prosthesis in the pocket of the bra and then gave it to me to try on.

I felt awkward at first because the bra was so heavy on one side due to the weight of the prosthesis. I put it on and then the fitter checked the fit. I was also instructed to put on the fitted knit shirt that I had brought with me to see how the new breast looked compared to its real mate. It was important that the contour of my figure looked symmetrical and that the size of the prosthesis matched the size of my natural breast. I looked into the mirror very intently. This was a very important purchase and required undivided attention. I also tried on the size eight and the size ten.

Mom gave her opinion about how each one looked to her. She wanted the fit to be absolutely perfect. The fitter was right when she had looked me over and sized me up originally. The size nine was the best fit. I tried it on again, this time with more confidence and a feeling of peace of mind. Mom looked at me just as she did when I was fitted for my wedding gown. She wanted everything to be exactly right. She wanted me to feel beautiful. And I did. Mom said, "You look whole again. I can sleep tonight." It was a good day for both of us.

I had a real appreciation for the fitter's skills. Being able to merely glance at my chest and know instinctively what size and shape of breast prosthesis I would look best in was truly amazing to me. I could better understand why they called these people "fitters." I also had an appreciation for the number of club members that had come before me based on the ease with which the fitter did this task and the volume of oversized shoe boxes that were in that closet, the Boob Closet. She cautioned me to wear my prosthesis regularly. She said that some women buy them but then put them away in the box and don't wear them. I found this surprising. Since that time, however, I have met a lot of other mastectomy patients who have experienced trouble with their prosthesis which has resulted in their switching to other brands or going without them completely. Small-busted women can have trouble with the prosthesis floating around in the pocket of their bra. Large-busted women like myself are sometimes troubled with the weight of the prosthesis. Because of its being made out of silicone and being solid matter, it doesn't give your skin an opportunity to breathe and can cause excessive sweating. I've had trouble with this myself and am busy with patenting what I hope will be a remedy for all mastectomy patients who suffer with the same problem. I definitely didn't want to have this very special item sitting at home in a box. I considered my prosthesis to be just as important as some people feel their American Express card is—I don't leave home without it!

Mom and I headed home to show Al how I looked. He was beaming when he saw me. He said, "Now which one has the Tony?" I pointed to the right side and said, "This one is the live one; the left side is the Memorex version." He could see that I had my confidence back. I stood taller now and walked without worrying that someone could tell that I had had a breast removed. I laughed to myself that night in bed about my preoperative trips to the shopping centers, searching for a fake boob on another woman. There was no doubt in my mind that I had probably seen quite a few breasts that were prosthetic versions of the real thing. These women had been to see some fitter at a mastectomy supply shop that carried breast forms.

Prostheses no longer look like jellyfish as they used to twenty-five years ago. They looked quite natural and when inside a bra could pass for the real thing without any trouble. There are times that Al still forgets about my surgery or forgets which side it was on and grabs my left side for a quick and risqué squeeze; when I don't respond, he realizes he's got the wrong side! I showed Jack, Al's brother, my prosthesis. He was very impressed and asked me if he could sleep with her sometime. You may have noticed that I referred to the prosthesis as *her*. That's because I decided to name my prosthesis. I had chosen a name even before I had chosen her. Her name is Betty—Betty Boob to be precise. I figured that choosing a prosthesis was similar to choosing a puppy. She was going to become a family member and would be spending a lot of time with me. Everywhere I went, Betty would also go. She deserved a name of her own. After all, she was to be my bosom buddy, right?

My friend Wanda, who lives in Virginia, brought me a special present when she came to visit me shortly after I had gotten Betty. It was a ceramic Christmas ornament that she had a crafter make for me. It was shaped like a baby bottle and had inscribed on it, "Betty Boob's First Christmas." Christmas was several months away but I chose not to wait for our tree to be up before I had this precious welcoming gift displayed. I hung it in our entryway and it became quite a conversation piece. I still enjoy looking at it.

About two weeks after I got Betty, I went back to We Fit and was fitted for a mastectomy bathing suit and a swimmer's breast prosthesis. Swimmer's prostheses are generally lighter in weight and are made of special foam that contains buckshot in the center of them to provide a little bit of weight. I had heard that when the manufacturing company first came out with the swimmer's model, it was only made out of Styrofoam and didn't function well. Apparently, when a woman got in the water, her prosthesis served as a floatation devise. Perhaps it would have been useful if she were learning how to swim or had fallen overboard while aboard ship, but for everyday use in a swimming pool, it was a loser. The next version that was released for sale was made of foam rubber. It was equally awful because it absorbed water just like a sponge. Not only would it pull the woman down in the water, but when she attempted to get out of the pool, her breast would be hanging at about waist level and would be spurting water. I can see these poor women now, saying, "Please excuse me while I go to wring out my breast." I was definitely fortunate that the trials and testing of this model were over. I was able to leave with a swimmer's model, size two. It works quite well, or should I rephrase that and say that *she* works quite well? Yes, she has a name too. Surely you can guess what Betty's partner's name is. Well for those of you that can't, her name is Esther. Esther Williams. What did you expect?

Since I have added Betty and Esther to our family tree I have had the opportunity to get information about some other prostheses that are also on the market. A friend of mine who had a mastectomy several years ago and is about my age sent me some literature and a videotape about a fairly new design of prosthesis that is becoming increasingly popular with women who have had a mastectomy and are average to small busted. The breast prosthesis sticks onto the woman's chest wall with Velcro. Yes, that's right—Velcro. A very creative person figured out how to use the same kind of adhesive that patients use for attaching ostomy bags to the skin and decided to try it out on women who don't want to worry with a prosthesis being in a pocket. Instead the woman applies a special adhesive tape that is nonirritating to the skin. The side of the tape that is exterior to the skin has Velcro on it. The inner portion of the breast form prosthesis also has Velcro on it that adheres to the Velcro strip on the tape. The woman just presses the prosthesis in place and voilà—she has herself a prosthesis that does not require a bra to keep it in place. From feedback that I have gotten from other women, this is a great model, but not very practical for large-busted women. The Velcro works to a point but the weight of the prosthesis for a woman of my bust size causes the skin to be pulled at the adhesive application site. That's okay. Betty and I are doing just fine anyway.

Al and I thought that if ever I changed my mind and I decided to get this stick on model, he would help me stick it on. Of course, we were not thinking about applying it using the techniques that were shown in the video tape. We thought that it would be great fun to have him stand back from me about ten feet, and, using the techniques of a baseball pitcher, throw it into place. Perhaps we could even keep score! Foul…strike one…Well, as I've said before, humor has been what has gotten us through many a bad day, and night.

I did put in a request to Al, however, for Christmas. I told him that this company also sold stick-on nipples. You could buy them in various skin tone shades as well as different diameter measurements. I told him that if he needed any gift ideas for me for the holidays, this could make a unique stocking stuffer!

Chapter 16

Returning to work was exciting but tiring. I expected my body to be ready to work my usual pace of sixty hours a week and it refused to cooperate.

It was marvelous to see everyone. My staff and coworkers were very glad to see me back and relieved that I was doing well. Working with so many women added a great deal to my support system, I think. Don't get me wrong, the men I work with and am very close to were certainly there for me when the chips were down, but the women I am close to and see each day could relate better to what I was going through. Of course each one of them, I'm sure, was hoping that she would not be the next one-out-of-nine to have the same experience that I had just gone through. It felt wonderful to get so many hugs. I didn't feel completely confident hugging people until I had my stuff and fluff replaced by Betty.

I also sent a lot of letters to family and friends during this six-week recovery period. I wrote special sentimental letters, thanking them for their support during the tough time, letting people know that I was a fighter and that I had no plans of giving up and letting the Big C get me. Holding on to optimism was key and sharing those thoughts was an uplifting experience for me. Under other circumstances I might not have sent such letters. Perhaps I would have considered it too corny or something. But it felt very appropriate to do so at the time. I wanted people to know that I appreciated them a lot, that their thoughtfulness and caring was a big part of my ability to recover so well. With their love I had hope. With their friendship I had a future. This had been an experience. I had truly been dealt a hand that showed me what I would get when I don't get what I want. But it also was a learning experience for me. I learned that life is precious, that my marriage could survive such an awful crisis, and that, with God's love and the support of friends and family, I could get through a crisis.

I also reflected frequently on the good fortune of being spared chemotherapy since my lymph nodes were negative. While I was getting well, our long time friend, John Cross, was getting sicker. He had had a craniotomy to attempt to remove a malignant brain tumor that proved to be only partially successful. While I gradually improved, John gradually got sicker. He and his wife, Pat, visited us frequently. We saw them quite a lot once he agreed to have his medical care transferred from the small-town hospital where they lived to Johns Hopkins Hospital. Though we were able to provide him the very best surgical and medical oncology treatment that could be offered, his gliosarcoma was a grade IV and would not respond to treatment. I visited his room daily. He and I had bonded like siblings. He always wanted to know how I was doing, what my blood-work results showed, how my x-rays looked. He told me that he wanted me to be "one hundred percent."

"If I have to lose some so that you can gain some, that's all right with me. I want you to be well again and stay well."

I watched this man slowly slip away . . . I watched his wife of more than twenty-five years become emotionally shattered and the rest of his family suffer. He died in the small town where he had lived nearly all of his life. I elected not to attend his funeral, even though my husband was a pallbearer. I feared that seeing him lying in a casket would be more than I could take. We had both battled cancer together. I was afforded the opportunity to be a survivor; he was not. Truly this was not due to lack of will power or desire, but solely due to the progression of his disease and God's will. I miss him to this day, but feel that somehow John is looking down on me and doing whatever is in his power to be my guardian angel.

In November of 1992, I was three and a half months into my recovery. Things were progressing along as scheduled until one morning when I was in the shower preparing to go to work when I felt a lump in my other breast. Oh no. This can't be happening to me. Why is this happening to me? The timing was awful as well, not that there is ever a good time to find a lump in one's breast. This particular morning was the day that the hospital was due for an inspection by the Joint Commission.

When I got to work I called to get an appointment with Charlie. I was already due for a mammogram at the end of that week, so I decided to leave the schedule as it was rather than change the x-ray to an earlier time. I wanted to get through this inspection first, then I'd deal with my own personal problems. If the lump was cancer, then it had just gotten there. If it was something benign, then it could wait anyway. I decided to use the inspection as a diversion from my medical problems. The inspection of the hospital's quality and utilization management programs went well. As soon as the surveyors were out the door, I was in the hands of the radiology folks, though, so that I could find out what the lump was. All that I could think about was that I feared Betty was about to have a roommate. I'd have two oversized shoe boxes with breast prostheses in them. I guessed I'd be calling them the Boobsy Twins.

Before long the mammogram was done. I was very nervous during the procedure. Once again I asked if my radiologist friend was available to be with me. He came into the room shortly after I made this request. Al was waiting out in the reception area for me. He had hives on his face, as usual. The female radiologist came into the room and said, "It looks like a cyst. I suggest that we make sure by doing an ultrasound exam. If it is, then it should probably be drained." A cyst…well that sounded good to me.

In the ultrasound room a much kinder machine was used. The mass that visualized on the screen did contain liquid. The next step was to drain the cyst. When Charlie had drained the cyst (which turned out to be the same one that had refilled and got a little bit larger this time), he stuck a tiny needle in it and—*poof*—it was gone. For some reason this time the procedure wasn't so simple. My breast was placed back in the mammography machine and converted into a waffle this time. The radiologist then inserted a needle. The pressure of the machine squeezing my breast caused the needle to automatically fill with fluid from the cyst. It was quite painful. I kept thinking that when she pulled the needle out, my breast would still be spouting fluid like a volcano that was erupting. It didn't, though. She confirmed on the ultrasound machine by taking before-and-after pictures that the cyst was completely empty now. I left the radiology suite with a sore chest but a smile on my face. Al was greatly relieved. Our radiologist friend had already been out to talk with him while I was having the aspiration done. It was just another dress rehearsal, I guess, but one that haunted me.

I saw Charlie just a few days later. He reviewed my radiology pictures and seemed satisfied that the problem was a cyst, but he added a little caution to his remarks. He told me that though the pathology report showed cystic fluid, that there was no guarantee that there weren't cancer cells present. He also recommended that if the cyst refilled again to have a lumpectomy done. He told me that I would now be on his close surveillance list of patients for the future. I told him that the fear of recurrence worried me. He appreciated my concern and discussed with me the option of having a prophylactic mastectomy done. This would be my choice, of course. If I started dreading each day because I worried about recurrence then it would be a smart thing to do. I decided to hold this option in reserve for now. Why have surgery if you don't absolutely have to?

Since that visit in November I have met several women who have chosen the preventive measure to keep them from worrying about the possibility of recurrence. Each seemed pleased with her choice. I decided to take the self-breast-exam route and try to think more optimistic thoughts. It certainly made me envious of that medical device that the doctor used *Star Trek*. Bones, as I believed he was nicknamed, would hold a little machine that looked like a small calculator over an ill person and, within a few seconds, the machine would chirp. He then would say, "It appears that this man is infected with a potentially deadly virus that is carried by a small insect that is only found on the planet Wolitble. I'll give him an injection of Smoglot and he will be well in a moment or two." Now wouldn't it be wonderful to personally own such a device? Who knows, maybe in the year 2050 there will be such a device; they'll be selling them a K-Mart as a blue-light special.

I didn't get to see my friend Lynda to show her how Betty and I looked as a team until Christmas week. We were over to their home for dinner and she and I went into their bedroom for a show-and-tell session. I showed her my incision first. She looked very intrigued with it and was impressed with the narrowness of my scar. I truly have excellent skin for good healing—a gene my father blessed me with. Then Lynda held my prosthesis. "Why, it feels just like a breast! This a amazing! See, I told you that you would do fine. This is merely an inconvenience, but it's not you. It's just flesh. Our Lillie is still here. Thank God!"

Laura became more inquisitive about my prosthesis too. One evening I found her in the bathroom holding it up to her chest as she evaluated her appearance in the mirror. "Laura, what are you doing with my breast prosthesis?" She glanced up, completely unstartled by my entering the bathroom and finding her in this odd situation. She said, "I was just wondering, if my breasts don't get as big as I want them to be, can any woman buy these or can you only get them if you've had a breast removed for cancer? I think that this thing is pretty neat. The boys would love it. Just look at how big I'd look if I wore yours!" I just shook my head and laughed. I assured her that her breasts would probably grow to a size that met her expectations and to not worry about it. But to answer her question, the answer was yes, any woman can buy these.

From the time that I had been diagnosed up until about six months after my surgery, a lot of people asked me whether or not I planned to have reconstruction done. I felt very uncomfortable with hearing this chronic question. I wasn't so much bothered by the fact that someone was asking as much as I was bothered by the way in which some people chose to make the inquiry. "Are you planning to have reconstruction? I had a friend who did and she is really happy with the results," or, "I know someone who had reconstruction. She had an awful time with it and had to have it undone, poor thing. You aren't looking to have that done, are you?" These questions didn't bother me in the least. But this one did: "You *are* going to have reconstruction, aren't you?" This was said in a way that implied that something was wrong with me if I didn't agree to have it done. On numerous occasions I was tempted to respond in a less-than-professional manner. Rather than saying my usual reply of, "Al and I have discussed it and I've opted not to have this done at this time and probably never will," I could have said, "No, I'm not. I've heard that you have had your face lifted and your nose fixed and obviously you didn't get your money's worth so I'm steering clear of plastic surgery for now."

I did give a lot of thought to reconstruction, though. It seemed that so many women had chosen to have it done. I was not a candidate for implants but was and still am a candidate for a tram-flap procedure. This procedure involves having your abdominal tissue and blood vessels moved from your belly to your chest. The result is that a breast mound is made that simulates a breast. Some women have even gone the whole nine yards and had a nipple reconstructed as well. The procedure is a lengthy one and recovery time is ten weeks. There is also a higher degree of infection with this procedure. Some women have been thrilled with the results. Others have not been happy at all. I have heard that women who have had reconstruction done simultaneous to their mastectomy are the least satisfied with the results. I personally think that this is because they are expecting too much. They awaken from surgery and don't see a breast missing; they see a mound of flesh that is trying to disguise itself as a breast. If the woman waits several months to have the reconstruction, then she has had some time to adjust to the loss and is more content with its simulated, internally attached replacement.

I based my decision on a multitude of things. First, I didn't want to undergo surgery that wasn't necessary and carried risk. Second, I wanted to know how important a facsimile version of a breast would be to my husband. He made it clear that it made no difference to him one way or the other and wanted me to base my decision on personal desire and not on him. Third, I asked Laura about her opinion. She was quite clear about her feelings about such surgery. She said, "No. I don't think that you should have this done. No one can replace your breast. It's gone. Moving your tummy tissue up to your chest doesn't give you a new breast. It simply covers up your scar by relocating skin and tissue that belongs someplace else. You look fine as your are. You should stay this way. Betty looks fine on you."

So my decision was made. I may change my mind some time in the future, but I doubt it. I also did fear that someday the other shoe would drop and I would have to have another mastectomy done. If this were to occur, I would not have achieved anything by having my left breast rebuilt. There would be nothing left to provide a reconstruction of the right side. So, we decided we'd all be content with Betty and continued to take advantage of the phantom-limb sensation that I had. This sensation would also be lost if I had the reconstruction. No more playing the game of "In search of the missing nipple"? Well then forget it!

I do respect the wishes and desires of other club members who have opted to utilize this option of reconstruction, though. It's marvelous that women nowadays have a choice. Knowing that I too have a choice and can utilize this same option in the future, if I so desire, is a good feeling.

Chapter 17

Traveling with a prosthesis is an adventure unto itself. At least the first few trips away from home are an experience and worth mentioning at this point in time. I had my first opportunity to travel with Betty on an overnight business trip during Thanksgiving week. I went to Philadelphia to do a consulting job at a large teaching hospital there. It was my first experience carrying heavy objects (my briefcase and a suitcase). I realized that my arm was not as strong as I thought it was. I felt doubly disadvantaged because my good arm also wasn't so good anymore due to having broken my right shoulder the year before my mastectomy. But I muddled through with the assistance of some Advil tablets.

When I got to my hotel room I discovered that, rather than my room having a king-sized bed as I had anticipated, it had two double beds. Normally I would have called down to the front desk and requested to be relocated into a room that had the size of bed that I was expecting, but this time I decided that I wouldn't bother. Who knows, maybe Betty had changed the reservations since she knew that she would be going on her first out-of-town adventure. So when I got ready for bed that night, I didn't put Betty in her oversized shoe box that she was usually stored in at home. Those boxes are not conducive to travel; the prosthesis storage box would have required its own suitcase just to bring it along on the trip. So I decided that just for the fun of it, I'd put Betty in the other double bed all by herself. If I had had access to a pair of stick-on eyes and a plastic fake nose, I would have put them on her and taken her picture. As it was, I was laughing myself to sleep anyway, thinking of how silly I was to put my prosthesis in her own bed. But it was fun. I was in the privacy of my own hotel room and all alone. The only way that anyone would know that I had done such a silly thing would be if the fire bells had rung and required a rapid evacuation of the building. Even under such circumstances, I think that I would probably grab my pocketbook and Betty before I considered leaving my room. Since there was no such emergency that night, Betty and I both rested well she in her own bed with pretty sheets, a blanket, and a gorgeous bedspread, and I in mine.

My next adventure with my prostheses was when we went to Disney World in April 1993. For this trip I also took my swimmer's breast prosthesis, Esther. I had purchased a new mastectomy bathing suit and was anxious to try out my new prosthesis in it. We spent our third day there at Typhoon Lagoon, which is a water park contained within Disney World. It has slides, swimming holes, a wave machine, and (my favorite) a relaxing ride that consisted of getting in an innertube and floating downstream for about a quarter of a mile. The ride was in Castaway Creek. This particular ride takes you in a giant circle around the park. I loved it. Esther seemed content enough as well. I rode around in the innertube for about an hour then got out to get some food.

It's funny how self-conscious you can feel when you're wearing something new, particularly if the new item is a breast. During the time that I was going to get food, walk around the park to watch the kids screaming their heads off in the wave-rider machine, and finally walk back to our staked-out area where we had left our towels and bags and such, I felt like people were looking at my chest. I was sure that this was all in my mind and that I was simply being overly self-conscious about my new bathing suit and prosthesis, but nonetheless I *felt* like people were staring at my chest with a look of puzzlement. It wasn't until later in the day when I went to the bathroom that I realized that my paranoia had a valid explanation behind it.

I got into the bathroom and waited in line for a few minutes before a stall became open. While waiting, I glanced over into the mirror to see how I looked in my new bathing suit and to assess how much sun I had gotten on my back. Esther had moved! That's right, moved. I don't mean to imply that she wasn't there anymore, but she had gotten herself twisted up somehow and was definitely not where she belonged. Rather than having the shape of a football and being symmetrically matched to my real breast, the prosthesis had dropped lower and turned itself from a horizontal position to a vertical one. No wonder people had been looking at me! Needless to say, when I got in the stall, I rearranged her back into position.

There was no reason to get upset about it. Actually, I found it sort of funny, and I learned the importance of making sure that a swimmers' prosthesis doesn't have a lot of room to roam and move about. That was what the problem was. When I was in the innertube with my arms in an odd position, the prosthesis had shuffled itself around and changed its position, thereby changing its shape. When we got back to our hotel room, I sewed the mastectomy bra pocket smaller to prevent Esther from moving around and changing her position in the future.

During that same week that we went to Disney World, I decided to write a special letter to someone. That special person was Erma Bombeck. I had read her article in *Red Book* about her experience with breast cancer and then saw portions of her article again in the *Reader's Digest*. I was really pleased that someone as professionally visible and famous as she would let the world know that she had become a club member several years ago. I wrote to her, telling her how much I admired her for coming forth and telling the world about her mastectomy surgery, and that I hoped that as a result of her having done so, other women would be inspired to go and get a mammogram too as well as do self breast exams. I also shared with her some of the funny experiences that had occurred with me during the period from diagnosis to treatment and thereafter.

The letter was sent inside an Easter card. This particular card was the perfect card for me to send to her. As a matter of fact, I had bought three of them and sent one to Charlie Yeo, one to my secretary Diane, and one to Bombeck. On the front of the card was an elderly woman with a large bosom, holding a basketfull of Easter eggs. It said, "This year I'm going to hide the Easter eggs where no one will ever think to look." Inside the card, it said, "In my bra."

Only three weeks after I sent Erma my letter, she wrote back. I was very flattered that she would take the time to respond and felt that much closer to someone else who had traveled the narrow and scary path required to become a breast cancer survivor.

She confirmed in my soul the value of humor as a great healer and that it is important not to be silent about the disease. The more people that know that there are a *lot* of club members out there, the quicker we will proceed to encourage more women to take advantage of preventive medical care. I hope it will also promote awareness of the government and other medical-research organizations so that adequate moneys are allocated to the treatment and prevention of breast cancer. It would be wonderful if we could finally find a cure and rid ourselves of this disease once and for all.

By the time we returned from our vacation in Disney World, it had been almost a year since my original biopsy had been done that had started me down the path of transformation. I could hardly believe that it had been almost a year. This also meant that I would soon be due for my annual gynecological exam as well as my first annual mammogram and visit to my surgeon. First came the gyn exam. No sweat—I wasn't at all concerned. I felt fine. I had no new menstrual problems. No problem. Right? Wrong.

While my gynecologist was examining me, he noted that my right ovary was slightly enlarged and very tender. I also had had blood work done the week before which showed an elevated testosterone level. Uh oh—not what I had expected. He said, "I think in view of your history of breast cancer that it would be wise to have some additional tests done to make sure that what we're seeing right now isn't ovarian cancer. I know that this is not what you want to hear, but I think that we need to exercise some caution here. I'll get you scheduled for a transvesical/transvaginal ultrasound procedure so that we can visualize the ovaries and see what the problem is."

This was definitely not what I had planned to hear. Anyway, when a man has his head in your crotch, the only thing that a woman wants to hear are positive things, not comments that sound negative. Oh well, I realized that I was about to undergo another experience.

When I got home that evening, I told Al the news. He said that he felt nauseated and had to leave the dinner table for a moment. Of course I prayed to God that whatever this problem was, it wouldn't be ovarian cancer.

Ovarian cancer makes breast cancer look like a simple case of acne. It is deadly. The survival rate is poor. I didn't want to think that I had just weathered the storm of breast cancer only to be swept away by its wicked stepsister, ovarian cancer.

My ultrasound procedure was two weeks later. For those of you who haven't had such a procedure done, it is somewhere in the same family with mammography. A large "wand" that looks like a dildo in disguise is inserted into the vaginal canal until it touches your tonsils. Now that might seem pleasurable to some, but not to me, especially since it is required for the patient to have a full bladder—a very full bladder. I was able to get the results right away, though. Hooray! It was an ovarian cyst! Now, normally I don't do college football cheers and cartwheels in the hall shouting, "Give a C, give me a Y, give me an S, give me a T," when I get news that I have an ovarian cyst, but compared to hearing the word "cancer" from the radiologist's mouth, I was absolutely thrilled! It was small and would be no problem.

Interestingly enough, there was no explanation as to why my testosterone was so high, though. Testosterone, of course, is a male hormone. Both sexes carry in their bodies some levels of both male and female hormones, but my testosterone was higher than the norm. I personally concluded that this was due to the environment that I worked in. When you are in the center of the political arena and the players you are contending with are male, it is useful to have an elevated testosterone level. I've read that some women who have had elevated testosterone levels had to compete with men in high executive positions. Perhaps that was what had happened to me. I really didn't care. I was simply relieved that I didn't have cancer. So were my family and friends.

A few weeks later, while I was in the shower, I felt a knot in my right breast. Ironically, it was in the same location where I had developed the breast pain the last year at this time, causing me to have the first mammogram done. It felt like an almond and was very hard. I was due for my annual mammogram in five weeks, so I decided just to watch it until then and not panic about it. It was probably just a cyst, no big deal. It remained consistently there, even during my periods, and by the time that it was the day to have my mammogram, it was slightly larger in size.

I had the mammogram on June 23rd in the morning. Al drove in from home to be with me during the procedure. He patiently waited out in the waiting room while I had the pictures taken. The radiologist felt the lump but was unable to visualize it on film. As I had heard said to me before, not all masses visualized on the mammography because, "Your breast tissue is very dense." I'm not sure if that is a compliment or a criticism, but I have always taken it as a compliment of sorts. That's because women who are young usually are the ones with dense breast tissue. Since the mammogram was inconclusive, I was taken into ultrasound to see if the lump visualized on film in there. I thought that it would, because I thought it was a cyst. That was wishful thinking on my part. No cyst visualized. The radiologist told me that she would have another doctor also look at the films but that they would probably be recommending a biopsy to be sure that this wasn't another primary tumor. My heart sank.

When I got dressed and went out to the waiting room, Al could see that I was not a happy camper. I told him the news. He kissed me and told me that no matter what the outcome, we'd be all right. I asked him to call my folks with the news. I was sticking to my bargain, which was to keep them informed, even though I really didn't want to give them any more bad news. I could already picture my mother's face with a droopy left eyelid due to the sudden development of a severe migraine headache when she heard this report. That's why I thought that it was best for Al to talk with them. He has a calming effect, somehow.

I already had an appointment with Charlie Yeo, my surgeon, on July 1. I didn't feel the need to try to move it ahead. It was less than a week away and would give the radiology department time to have my films reread by another doctor. It would also give me time to collect myself and think about the possible consequences of the next step. This was not what I had pictured as the events surrounding my first anniversary as a breast cancer survivor. Just when I thought it was over, or better said, just when I had *hoped* that it was over, I realized that it wasn't. And if this was to be merely another dress rehearsal, then how many more dress rehearsals would there be in my future? Would there never be a true closure to my experience with breast cancer? I realized that the answer was already known to me but had been strategically pushed far to the back of my brain. No, there would never be *complete* closure. Once breast cancer has touched you, you are always watchful for its return.

I think that this is one of the reasons why women often wait a year or even longer before they start attending breast cancer support-group meetings. They have the support they need while going through the actual crisis of receiving the diagnosis and going through the surgery, even chemo and radiation. But once a year of time has passed and the crisis is over, there is that part of a woman's brain that chronically fears the potential return of the disease, or the visitation of one of its relatives like ovarian cancer, lung cancer, or bone cancer. I've seen it on the faces of women that I've talked with who were members of support groups. On this particular night I saw a very clear picture of what a frightened woman looked like who was afraid that cancer had returned. I found this woman staring back at me from my bathroom mirror.

Once again, my family and coworkers were there to support me. Marge, one of my staff, was especially supportive during the week between my mammogram and when I actually got to see my surgeon. Bryanna, another one of my staff, had the opportunity to see Charlie during that week and, with my permission, gave him a capsulated version of what was going on with me. He was prepared for a nervous Nelly in the exam room. My secretary Diane was definitely in a state of denial about the whole thing. I didn't talk much about it because I was afraid that she would cry, and if she cried, I would also be standing in a bucket of tears right beside her. Scott was also very supportive and wanting all of this awfulness that seemed to keep happening to me to go away.

My appointment with Charlie was during my lunch hour. I had picked up my mammography and ultrasound films from radiology so that he could see them too. He already had in my file a printed copy of what the radiologists' reading of the films had shown. He spent a lot of time examining me and of course focused intently on the hard lump that had appeared only six weeks ago. His advice was the same as that of the radiology physicians. Biopsy was the only way for us to know for sure what it really was. He said that he would schedule me for an open excisional biopsy under local anesthesia with some IV sedation. It would be scheduled in about ten days or so.

I called Al and told him of the plans for outpatient surgery. The procedure was to be done during our vacation week. I'm sure that if I had told Charlie that I was to be on vacation, he would have booked me for later in the month, but I didn't want to wait. I wanted to get this over, so that I knew what I was dealing with. Laura was distressed when I told her that I had to have another biopsy. She said, "Tell them that you've had enough done. I don't want you losing the other breast. One is enough." She was without humor that evening. She looked serious and acted serious. I caught her staring at me frequently while we sat together in the living room, watching a movie on the television. I don't know what she was thinking. Quite frankly, I was afraid to ask.

Al and I talked a lot that weekend. That was the weekend of the Fourth of July. The last year at that time, he was consoling me about the mastectomy surgery that I was scheduled to have when we returned from our vacation in Maine. Now he was consoling me about the possibility of having another biopsy. I was trying to brace myself for the results, no matter which way the outcome went, though. I also explained to him that Charlie might end up doing a lumpectomy with the biopsy. If so, my remaining breast might actually be a little smaller than it was presently. If the biopsy was negative and the breast was smaller I would need to get a prosthesis a size or two smaller than what I already had. Betty was a size nine. She was definitely a pretty hefty girl. Though she came with a two-year warranty, she didn't come with a trade-in policy. I doubted that she would be a very salable item in a yard sale, either. Perhaps she would draw a good crowd to a yard sale, though. You know, like tires do. Maybe I could run an ad in the newspaper in order to sell her. It could say:

> *For Sale to a good and loving home. One left-sided, externally-worn silicone breast prosthesis. Her name is Betty. Excellent condition. Only nine months old. Seeking a woman who is in need of a left breast. Still under her two-year warranty. Also still a virgin. Please call present owner for an agreeable time to see her and make offer if interested.*

Well, that could be an option, depending on the outcome of my biopsy. I figured that there were three possibilities:

1) The procedure would require an excisional biopsy with little tissue removed. The results would be negative. No further changes would be needed.

2) The procedure would involve a portion of the breast being removed which would result in Betty being larger than her flesh-and-blood mate. If so, then Betty might have to be put away in my hope chest as a souvenir of the past and a replacement in perhaps a size eight or seven would be purchased.

3) The biopsy would be positive and I'd be in search of the Boobsy Twins as my prosthetic replacements.

Oh, yes, I guess there could have been a fourth possibility—cancel the biopsy and arrange to take the next space shuttle to Mars. That didn't seem very plausible, though.

On July 6, I returned to work after the holiday weekend and received a call from my surgeon's secretary that my surgery had been scheduled for July 14th during the following week. The 14th. Does that ring a bell? It did for me. That was the same date that I had had my mastectomy just one year ago. I asked myself questions. What does this mean? Should I start reserving operating room time for next July 14th? Is this a sign that surgery was going to be an annual event?

I called Al at home and gave him the information about the date and time for the surgery. I waited until I got home to talk with my folks and let them know the specifics. My mother sounded very distressed that this surgery would be on the same day as last year's surgery. It felt like an omen. I tried very hard not to think too much about it, but it was not easy. I also decided to tell only a few people at work about it to avoid creating a panic and have rumors running rampant that I was about to go six feet under.

Since I was going to be receiving IV sedation this time, I wanted to touch base with Dr. Pasternak who was the medical director of the outpatient center. He was also an anesthesiologist. I connected up with him later in the week and told him that I would be a patient in his neck of the woods the following week and inquired as to who was scheduled for that day as the "sandmen" for anesthesiology. He told me that he was one of the physicians on that day but would be happy to arrange for one of the female anesthesiologists to be with me for the procedure. I requested that he be with me. He was someone I trusted and knew fairly well.

He was concerned that, because I would be awake during the procedure with drugs in me to control pain, I might feel self-conscious about his seeing me topless. I assured him that my priority was my health and not my modesty.

Anyway, since my mastectomy last summer, I wasn't as shy as I used to be. Figuratively speaking, I'm only *half* as shy.

Al once again had the unpleasant chore of alerting our friends and family members about the new development. Prayers were offered up from everyone and from all denominations of faith. That was a very reassuring feeling for me. Al had a very positive outlook about it and felt that perhaps the tide had finally changed and this time the news would be good for me, for us. I wanted to think positively too, but found it harder this time. I didn't lose my sense of humor, though, and we spent a lot of time joking about Betty possibly being replaced with a slightly smaller model and what we would name twin prostheses if I needed them.

To further complicate my parents' lives, Dad was informed by his physician that his PSA level was high. This is a special blood test that can help to detect abnormalities of the prostate gland in men. It is used as a marker for possibly detecting prostate cancer. This meant that he was also going to be biopsied. His was scheduled two days after mine.

I was off on vacation for two days before my surgery was to be done. I probably would have been better off working, but I took the time off anyway. We just didn't do the things that we had originally planned to do during that time, like enjoy ourselves.

The day before my surgery, several of my staff at work sent me a beautiful bouquet of flowers to wish me well. I also received several cards in the mail that day and a lot of phone calls that night offering prayers that my results would be good ones this time. My surgery was scheduled for 12:15 P.M. on a Wednesday. I asked that my folks not try to come over because they had just picked up my brother's family from the airport after midnight on Tuesday. The family had flown in from Japan to spend their vacation time with all of us. Laura was over on my parents' farm with them as well. So it was just Al and I that day at the hospital together. It certainly felt like a *déjà vu* experience, being in the same day surgery suite, seeing the same faces that I had seen one year before, putting on the hospital gown, feeling my heart race.

While the nurses prepped me, Al waited out in the waiting room. He received a surprise visit from Marge and Scott and they gave him a card signed by many members of my department wishing for me all good things. Their timing was impeccable. Once I was prepped, Al was then allowed to rejoin me and stayed with me until it was time for me to go into surgery. He said that he was fine but had the beginnings of hives on his face.

A female anesthesiologist came in and talked with me about my anesthesia history problems that I had experienced in the past and said that she and another woman would be in the operating room with me. I was too nervous to ask about Dr. Pasternak, though I had seen him a few moments before and suspected that he preferred to have these female folks be with me during the unveiling part of the preparation where the doctor has the patient topless for a few seconds until the surgical drapes are applied to the surgical site.

Charlie came in to see me at this point and was his usual cheerful and calming self. He asked me how I was doing and I responded by saying that I was as nervous as a prostitute in church. Within minutes I was being walked into the operating room. I gave Al a big kiss, exchanged I-love-you's, and was escorted into the chilly room where the deed was to be done once again. The harder I tried not to shake, the more I shook. I felt embarrassed to be so frightened but was definitely more frightened than embarrassed.

I also had a fear, silly at it may seem, that while under the influence of drugs (conscious sedation) I'd talk and say heaven knows what about whom. Maybe I'd feel some compelling need to describe details about my sex life with my husband. Maybe I'd be mean to people that were trying to take care of me and help me into the operating room. I had been with my father on several occasions when he was awakening from general anesthesia and he was most unpredictable about what he would do or say. On one occasion he was very nasty and cursed a lot. (To be specific, he wanted someone to give him his teeth so he could bite his surgeon in the rear end!) On another occasion, while awakening from anesthesia, he turned into a Casanova and told the recovery room nurse that she had beautiful breasts and asked if he could touch them. I was shocked. All of this behavior was very out of character for him. Who knew what I might say or do under the influence of similar drugs. Remember, I would be seeing all of these faces again, and on a frequent basis, because I worked at the place where my medical care was being provided.

Once on the operating-room table, Charlie drew a circle around the location of the lump and I was then placed in a horizontal position on the table and strapped down. I realized that I was truly about to lose total control of the situation and had to place my faith in the Lord and the health care providers who surround me. I heard the anesthesiologist say to Charlie as he exited the room to go scrub up that my blood pressure was very high. That was the last thing that I remembered.

When next I opened my eyes, I was in the recovery room and my throat felt sore. I struggled to focus on the clock on the wall and realized that several hours had passed. I then knew that I must have been put all the way to sleep. Al appeared. A nurse appeared. So did the anesthesiologist, director of nursing, medical director, and several other people, each inquiring how I felt, each reassuring me that the procedure was over and I was okay now. True, I was physically okay, but what was it that was taken out of my breast?

Shortly thereafter, Charlie appeared. Calming, reassuring, he said that he decided to put me under anesthesia because I was very upset during the procedure. I didn't remember any of the procedure, though. I asked if I had talked at all and he wittingly teased me and said, "Oh yes, you talked a whole lot." Then he smiled and shook his head no and said that I hadn't talked at all. I'll probably never really know if I did or didn't. Hopefully, if I did talk, I spoke about the weather.

Charlie said that the mass was fairly large but that the color of the tissue looked good and that he felt hopeful this time but didn't want us to hang our hat on this preliminary news. Last year we had thought that everything was okay and got a bad surprise in the end. He wanted me to call him in five days to get the path report. Five days sounded like an eternity to me.

An hour or so later, I was being escorted out of the hospital via a wheelchair and Al picked me up at the door. Once home, I lay down to rest and put an ice bag on my bandages. Charlie had instructed me to wear my bra for a week around the clock to provide support to the surgical site. This meant that Betty would be sleeping in the bed with Al and me. It was strange. I thought that it would be uncomfortable having three pounds of silicone in the bed with me, but it wasn't. I found myself sleeping in positions that I hadn't been able to assume since I had my mastectomy. I hadn't even realized that I had developed different sleeping positions with my left arm until that moment. It made me feel melancholy for the flesh that had been there prior to Betty's arrival.

Though the weekend was busy with my brother's family with us from Japan, it was hard not to constantly think about what the verdict would on Monday afternoon. I was at the hospital on Friday to be with my father during his prostate biopsy procedure and stopped upstairs to see Charlie's secretary, Tracy, for a moment. She advised me of his schedule for Monday and that the best time to call would probably be after 1:30 P.M. I also left a funny card for him with a personal note thanking him for getting me through this crisis to date and telling him that I would be back in touch with him on Monday afternoon for the verdict. The card had a cartoon drawing of a man and woman sitting in a ski-lift chair. As they were traveling in the ski-lift chair, they passed a sign that said, "PLEASE KEEP YOUR TIPS UP." The female skier, who was very well endowed, was sitting in the chair holding her robust boobs up with her hands. The man in the chair with her looked at her and said, "Excuse me, miss, I believe the sign refers to one's skis . . ." Inside, the card said, "Seeing you is always an uplifting experience." I felt confident that Charlie would enjoy that card.

Monday finally arrived. I was in Reading, Pennsylvania, because I was shopping with my sister-in-law at the outlet stores there. My energy level was still low, but I was determined to shop with her. They were only home from Japan once a year and it was their vacation time. It was my vacation time, too. I kept watching the clock. We were heading home and had reached Lancaster when the clock reached 1:30 P.M. We had stopped to eat lunch, so I called from a pay phone to Charlie's office. My heart was beating so fast I felt like it could have leaped out of my chest and run around the block without me. It was unfortunately very noisy as well because of people bustling in and out of the restaurant. I felt for a moment like turning into Miss Piggy and decking anyone who laughed out loud or spoke loudly while walking by me. I thought to myself that this was how a crazed maniac must feel right before he goes into a public place, takes out a semiautomatic gun, and blows away anything that moves. Where were those kind of lunatics when you needed them? I certainly didn't want to kill anybody, but probably waving a large gun around might have gotten the room quieter, which was all that I desired.

I got a line through to Charlie's office and realized that the voice on the other end was not that of his secretary. His secretary was not in at the time and she told me that he was still waiting for my path report results. That would mean more waiting. She recommended that I call back in an hour.

I went into the restaurant to join my sister-in-law and niece. We ordered our food. I could hardly concentrate on the menu to make a selection, much less eat what the waitress brought me. She probably could have served me a section of innertube and I would have eaten it about the same way I ate the turkey platter that I ordered. My brain was in oblivion and my taste buds had traveled with my brain to keep it company. It was 2:30 P.M. when we were nearing the completion of our meal. I excused myself and went out to use the pay phone again.

At last the verdict was in, and the news told to me was good news this time! No cancer! It was a benign mass of fibrocystic tissue. I didn't know who the pathologist was who had dictated the report, but I loved him. I immediately called Al at home and told him the good news. He must have told me that he loved me five times. I then scampered back into the restaurant and went over to our table. "It's okay. It's benign." I then broke into tears. Mary threw her arms around me and hugged me tightly. The crisis had passed once again. The dress rehearsal was over.

A few months after my surgery, I was fitted once again for a new prosthesis. Enough tissue had been removed from my right breast to make me a cup size smaller, so Betty required a downsizing. I sent Betty, size nine, to a local hospital to be given to a future club member who lacked health insurance. I am sure she is in a good home. I replaced her with a Betty size 8.

But how many more dress rehearsals would there be? None? Three? Ten? How can a breast cancer survivor distinguish a dress rehearsal from the real thing? There is no way. It goes with the diagnosis, I suppose. Sure, some women may deal better with the fear of recurrence than others, but I'd wager money that there is no breast cancer patient that doesn't live with some degree of anxiety that cancer will return, either in the other breast or in some other organ. That's why it's important to maintain your support systems that you have and utilize them when you need them. If you think that you're being a pain and bothering your friends or family, just remember the odds. One out of nine women develop breast cancer sometime in their life. It is predicted that this number will be one in eight by 1994.

While friends or family are helping you, they are also helping themselves—helping themselves get acquainted with breast cancer and its treatment and pitfalls. Because there is a strong possibility that one of those people is going to need your support in the future. During the twelve months after my mastectomy, five of my friends underwent breast biopsies and experienced first hand the feeling of a dress rehearsal. One additional friend underwent a breast biopsy and was not as fortunate as the others; she too became a breast cancer survivor club member, having had her mastectomy only a few weeks ago. She is our daughter's own godmother.

What can we do about this disease that has touched so many of us and so many of our friends? We can seek out the good things that have resulted from these experiences. When you are going through it, it can be hard to find the good but it's important to look within ourselves and seek it out. The roses do smell more fragrant now than they did in the past. Our family ties are more precious than we had realized before. Life is precious and has not been given to us to be wasted. That's why I became a nurse, I guess, so that I could help people get well again and get on with their business of living.

It's scary to think that during 1992, there were one hundred eighty thousand women diagnosed with breast cancer. One woman died of breast cancer every twelve minutes. There have been nights that I have lain in bed, unable to sleep due to so many things being on my mind. As I watched the clock slowly tick away one night, I realized that over a period of a little more than a half an hour, three fellow club members somewhere in the United States had succumbed to this deadly disease. That's truly a startling thought. It's important for those of us who are club members and have been blessed to be among the survivors of the disease to speak out to encourage preventative care. We need to get involved with breast cancer support groups and help those women who have been diagnosed after us to deal with the emotional roller coaster they are riding on. We need to learn from those who have been diagnosed and treated before us as to how to deal with the anxiety and fear of possible recurrence within ourselves. We need to promote breast cancer education in our community so that more women will do self breast exams and have annual physicals and mammograms. No, that won't reduce the number of women diagnosed each year; actually, it might increase the number, but it will reduce the numbers of deaths due to this disease. Early detection can, most of the time, equate to a higher survival rate. It's also important to get involved politically and promote and support bills in Congress that are directed toward research dollars going exclusively toward breast cancer research as well as toward mammography and treatment for women who otherwise would not receive care at all.

Since my mastectomy surgery, I have gotten involved with local breast cancer support groups, including those that are available through network computers. I feel that I am helping others and also benefiting myself. When I reached my one-year anniversary as a breast cancer survivor, I was eligible to sign up to be a Reach to Recovery volunteer. This gave me an opportunity to see patients who have undergone mastectomy surgery at Hopkins and talk with them about their emotional feelings and help them through those early days of learning to live without a breast. It gave me a unique opportunity to blend my nursing skills with that of my mastectomy experience while simultaneously working with health care professionals that I know and respect.

Reach to Recovery has made some positive changes over the last few years and now has volunteers available for visits before surgery as well as afterward. It is a pleasure for me to volunteer my evening hours in this way and I feel that I will be a stronger person for it.

My Avon representative Judy has given me Avon sample products to include in the mastectomy supplies and American Cancer Society literature that I provide to women who have undergone a mastectomy. Avon has a national breast cancer crusade campaign that they began in September of 1993. They are selling pink ribbon pins; these pins are a symbol of breast cancer awareness. All of the money raised through these sales goes toward breast cancer education. I wear my pin with pride and am seldom without it on my clothing. I always make a point of wearing it when I go on my Reach to Recovery hospital visit. The sample Avon items that Avon provides me as an Reach to Recovery volunteer further exemplify Avon's commitment to women. Avon wants all women to feel beautiful. During a medical crisis such as breast cancer, when a woman may be doubting her femininity, Avon is there for her as well.

My goal is to be like the Maytag repairman. I'm sure that you've all seen those commercials on television about him. He sits in an office, alone, very bored, waiting for the phone to ring. If the phone rings, then it means that someone needs his expert assistance in repairing a Maytag washing machine. In the commercial, the Maytag repairman's phone doesn't ring. Presently I receive several calls a week from various people who need to talk about breast cancer. It might be someone at the Reach to Recovery office who needs me to see a patient in the hospital or it might be a friend who knows someone who has just been diagnosed with breast cancer and is seeking advice about treatment or the disease. That's why I'd like to be like the Maytag repairman; I want to be bored with the job because there will be no one out there who needs my help, my support. I want to see breast cancer become a part of medical history for my future grandchildren and great-grandchildren to read about in textbooks and not know about from personal experience. When the phones across the country that are linked to breast cancer support groups, coalition organizations, breast cancer treatment centers, cancer associations, and Reach to Recovery stop ringing, then we can all sleep well at night, knowing that this disease has finally been stopped dead in its tracks. Our mothers, daughters, granddaughters, spouses, and friends will sleep better in the future, too.

Chapter 18

More time passed and soon it was once again time for my next mammogram. My first real annual mammogram was in June 1994. Why do I describe it as "real"? Because all the mammograms I had to date were due to having developed something that required a mammogram to determine its cause. This mammogram was different; this time I had no lumps, no known signs of any problems. It had been a year since my last films were taken, which were done right before the lumpectomy on my remaining breast.

I felt somewhat nervous about having this x-ray taken, primarily because I had only had my breasts placed in the vice machine due to having symptoms that something was wrong. I guess you could say that it was what scientists call a trident effect; if your association with something is always a negative association, then even when you'd like it to be positive, your stomach remembers the negative association and makes you feel like you want to throw up.

Nevertheless, though I went into the mammography suite feeling butterflies in my stomach, I still had a sense of confidence that this time I would be told what I had longed to hear: "Looks great! No abnormalities found." That wasn't what I was told, though. After having three different views taken, the technician told me that the radiologist had requested additional pictures because she saw something.

How could this be? After several more x-rays were taken, I was led to the sonogram room where an ultrasound was done. The objective was to determine if the masses (yes, I said mass<u>es</u>) were cysts (containing fluid) or tumors (solid in nature). Needle aspiration was attempted. After approximately an hour and a half, I realized that I was in the early stages of having another experience.

Though I already had a routine appointment with my surgeon for a checkup, the radiologist recommended that I not wait three weeks to see him and instead insisted that I call him to get an appointment sooner than that. In the meantime, the radiologists very kindly made arrangements to dictate a report about the x-ray results and fax them to Charlie's office. My anxiety as well as that of my family and coworkers once again was heightened in anticipation. It was hard to concentrate on work, but I knew that this would be my best therapy—to stay focused and occupied until I had more information about my situation. The radiology report looked ominous, though, and my husband and I discussed the serious possibility of another surgery.

Al accompanied me to my doctor's appointment to see Charlie Yeo. Al waited in the visitor's area while I went in to get the verdict. I couldn't stop shaking. In a matter of moments Charlie was there with me. He could see how nervous and upset I was. He reviewed the films with me, examined me, and then we talked. He discussed with me that my body seemed prone to grow things in undesirable places, like my breasts. It would be necessary to determine if these masses were benign or malignant, which would, at a minimum, mean another open biopsy. Then we discussed what I felt would probably be the inevitable anyway—a second mastectomy. He spoke to me calmly and compassionately, realizing how emotionally difficult all of these experiences to date had been. We discussed the positive aspect of choosing this option, and I told him that I didn't want to keep coming to his office every summer to be told that my remaining breast had grown something again that needed to be removed. Being whittled away to nothing, eventually, was not the route I wanted to choose. I told him that I agreed that the best option for me, whether these tumors were benign or malignant, was to have my new Betty get a roommate. (I didn't have the courage to say the word *mastectomy*.) I then asked him to talk with my husband. Charlie very carefully asked me if I wanted him to bring Al here to the exam room or if I wanted him to talk with Al alone. I pondered this question for about fifteen seconds, though it felt like five minutes. My choice was to have the men discuss this matter without my being within hearing distance. Charlie left me to get dressed while he spoke with Al in a secluded part of the waiting area.

About five minutes later, they both appeared before me. Al told me that the only thing that mattered to him was that I was with him, here on this earth, for as long as possible, no matter what it took. Tears flowed down my face as if someone had turned on a faucet behind each eyeball. The realization of all of this had really just hit me.

Charlie asked us both to ponder this decision over the weekend and call him Monday to let him know if I still wanted to take this surgical route. We did discuss it a lot over the weekend, and we also talked with my parents and our daughter about it. Everyone, including our daughter, to my surprise, felt that it was the very best option for me to go with. Our daughter, Laura, now age fourteen and two years older that she was with my first mastectomy, told me that she felt relieved because she had been worrying that the cancer might come back. She also said that I looked great with my new Betty and that whomever I chose to be Betty's roommate would look equally good on me.

The decision had been made, and on Monday I called Charlie's office and confirmed a date for my surgery. It would be two weeks later. Once again, I implemented every support system that I had. My parents, especially my mother, were coping much better this time than before. Maybe my mother realized that she could stop worrying about recurrence of breast cancer. If the masses were cancer, they would be gone; if they were benign, then we wouldn't have to worry about their turning into something bad later on, or my body producing more tumors, since there would be virtually no breast tissue for them to grow in anymore.

It was very important to focus on the positives and not the negatives. And it was equally important to keep a sense of humor at all times. Prayers were being sent up by hundreds of people. Mary, my roommate from nursing school, had even arranged for special masses to be held for me in her church as well as in a convent on the West Coast (and gee, I'm not even Catholic). My staff kicked into gear just as they had before and I felt confident that they would hold down the fort in my absence.

On June 27, 1994, I went through my last stage of transformation and my second mastectomy was performed. I had wanted to wear a tassel on my nipple when I went into the operating room suite, but worried that those people who would be in there assisting with the surgery, whom I didn't know personally, might find it too bizarre. Instead, I told my surgeon in front of everybody what I had planned to do and then opted not to. Heaven only knows what those nice people thought. To be safe, Charlie also removed lymph nodes from my axillary area as well as the chest wall.

The following morning I was scheduled for release. Charlie came in to check my incision shortly before I was to be released. As he removed my binder and dressings to expose the incision, Al looked on with an expression of complete acceptance of my body. Charlie then said to me, "Your chest looks like my new two-year-old daughter's chest. We've recently adopted a little girl from Russia. We feel that having gone overseas to bring her back to the States to live with us that so that she can be part of our family is like giving her the chance to be reborn. So is the case for you, Lillie; you now look as if you have been reborn." I don't think that a more appropriate or thoughtful expression of caring and acceptance could have been offered to me that day. It made me feel accepted. It made me feel special. It made me feel whole.

Nine days later, I returned to see him and get my hemovac drains pulled out and receive information about my pathology results. The masses contained within the breast were found to be in a precancerous state and the lymph nodes were negative. Al was thrilled as were my parents and friends. We immediately began adding to our list of all of the advantages of having the second surgery done: No more annual mammograms! No more fretting about the results of a mammogram! I could be whatever size I wanted to be now—I could look like Dolly Parton one day and Peter Pan the next!

There were other things that would require some time to adjust to. I worried about how this loss would affect our sex life. (Al didn't worry at all, but of course I did.) Al told me that since there is a proven theory that if you lose one of your senses (like your sense of sight or sense of hearing) that your other senses become more intensified. Therefore, he believed that if you lose one of your erotic zones, that either you develop a new one someplace else or your remaining ones become more intensified. He said that it was his job to prove this hypothesis. So when I reached five weeks post-op, he took me away to the Pocono Mountains to prove his theory. I now call him Professor Shockney. If it were possible to give him some type of honorary award, I would. In my opinion, having proven this hypothesis, I think that he should get a Nobel Prize at the very least.

Other good things have resulted from my experiences with breast cancer, too. I received in the mail a catalog from a company called Jodee. This company is known nationally for making mastectomy bras and other garments exclusively for women who have had breast surgery. Contained in the catalog was a letter written by the president and founder, Buddy Greenberg. In this letter was information about the company—information that explained that they had been in business since 1971 and their commitment was to serve the special needs of almost a million women who have had breast surgery. They seek out opportunities to share ideas and experiences with consumers, health care professionals, physicians, nutritionists, husbands, boyfriends, parents, and children, all of whom have relationships with women who have been confronted with breast cancer professionally or personally. The letter itself was an open invitation to its readers to write or call Mr. Greenberg personally and share any information that people wished to, whether it was related to ideas about new and special needs someone has or simply to express their opinions about the Jodee garments they have been wearing.

I chose to take Mr. Greenberg up on his offer and write to him. Within my letter was a suggestion about the potential use of a special kind of fabric that I had been using as an additional liner in the pocket of my mastectomy bras that helped to reduce the amount of perspiration that the prosthesis causes. I also told him about this book that I had written and that because his products are truly superb, I had elected to list his company in the resource chapter of my book.

On the same day that Mr. Greenberg received my letter, he called to talk with me. I felt very honored that he would take the time to do this. I could tell by the sound of his voice and his compassion for women who are breast cancer survivors that he was truly a special person. We talked about my suggestions in my letter. We had another conversation two days latter and at that time he asked me to come as his guest to visit him and his "professional family."

I was thrilled to be invited and made arrangements to go to Hollywood, Florida, where the Jodee Institute is located. I met with Buddy Greenberg and his vice-president, Louise Rose, who is also a breast cancer survivor. This was truly a unique and special opportunity because I was able to see first hand the wide variety of products that they make. It was amazing to watch rows and rows of sewing machines busily creating special mastectomy bras for women of various sizes and shapes. When you see such an operation in progress, it makes you stop and pause a moment about just how many breast cancer survivor club members there really are and how many more will be coming along behind me to also join the club.

I had the wonderful good fortune to be professionally fitted for prostheses and bras while I was there. Having been fitted now three different times, I can say without hesitation that Jodee has it down to an art how to properly fit a woman for prostheses as well as mastectomy bras. It requires special training, a keen eye, and a lot of tender loving care, compassion, and sensitivity.

I couldn't help but wonder how Mr. Greenberg got into this business that had been established nearly a quarter of a century ago. He explained to me that a friend of his mother had undergone a total radical mastectomy in 1964. She had battled with having to make do with her bras that she had worn for years prior to having had breast cancer and that these garments weren't working out for her at all. She wasn't alone with this problem. It was, however, during a time that women didn't talk about their surgeries much less discuss the difficulties that they were experiencing regarding their undergarments. It is a known fact, however, that if a woman doesn't feel comfortable in her clothes and, even more importantly, confident in her appearance, it will be evident in every aspect of her life. It lowers a woman's self-esteem. It prevents her from being able to restore her soul, to move on beyond the point where cancer has taken her, and on to the point of beginning her true emotional recovery. Mr. Greenberg could see this problem because of his dear family friend. She asked him if he could make her a bra that would help her feel more confident about her appearance; one that would be comfortable, practical, and provide her the confidence she so badly needed restored. He did exactly that. Mr. Greenberg continued to make these garments at no charge and gave them to friends and friends of friends.

In 1971, Mr. Greenberg read about Terese Lasser and her work with the Reach to Recovery Program developed with the American Cancer Society. The two of them met and Mr. Greenberg offered to contribute his design to the Reach to Recovery Program. Ms. Lasser said, "We are a nonprofit organization and therefore cannot accept your offer." She did, however, urge him to go into business, because she had traveled to thirty-seven countries looking for a functionally comfortable design and he was the only one who had it. Thus, the Jodee bra company was founded.

Mr. Greenberg developed a special bra to be used immediately after surgery as well as after the woman's discharge from the hospital, since the immediate restoration of the woman's natural silhouette is her first step toward her recovery. This soft feminine stretch-lace lounge bra with a convenient front closure and built-in stretch pockets accommodated the fluff prosthesis given to the patient by the Reach to Recovery volunteers. The bra replaced the need to use safety pins that could cause a problem.

Mr. Greenberg, through Jodee Bra Company, has contributed to the American Cancer Society for their Reach to Recovery Program over three million dollars in samples of products and price-reduced products over the last twenty-four years. In 1973 alone, his company provided, free of charge, three thousand mastectomy lounge bras for women who had just undergone mastectomy surgery. He truly is the pioneer of the mastectomy garment business and continues to provide support to organizations whose mission is like his own—to help women to have their confidence restored about their appearance, to help them progress along their road to recovery, and to complete the necessary research to eventually prevent breast cancer from attacking other women in the future. Mr. Greenberg told me that a primary mission of Jodee is to ensure a woman's privacy. That's why he developed a mail-order catalog business for his company. He knows that women don't enjoy going to be fitted for prostheses and bras because they have to expose their bodies to strangers. Many women even feel uncomfortable going into a store that specializes in mastectomy supplies because they don't want to be recognized by others that they have lost one or both breasts. There are many women who have chosen never to confide in anyone other than their spouses that they've even had breast cancer. There are, as a result, many women who have never been fitted for prostheses or mastectomy bras. They are still wearing their husbands' socks in their bras. Part of my mission now is to reach more of these women and make sure that they are given information about the options they have to be properly fitted while maintaining their privacy, thereby restoring their self-esteem that they had before breast cancer robbed them of it.

During my visit with Mr. Greenberg and his staff, we talked about the direction that medical research is starting to take regarding breast cancer prevention. He and his executive staff were very eager to learn about and financially contribute to worthy organizations that are taking the steps necessary to prevent breast cancer. We talked at great length about the company's contributions being spent on true prevention. I could not help but admire such a man who, in essence, says, "I want to support an organization that is working on true breast cancer prevention so that someday I can be put out of business." All too often business executives are only interested in how they can benefit from such work. It was refreshing to hear such a firm sense of commitment for the betterment of women's health.

Getting breast cancer was one of the worst experiences of my life; it also has been one of the best experiences because of all that I have gained from it. People ask me questions that constantly reaffirm positive beliefs. Questions like:

> *Question: How has your marriage been since your mastectomies? How is your sex life?*
> *Answer: My marriage was good before, but now it's even stronger. I have always been happy with our sex life and it, too, has improved despite the loss of both of my breasts. If a woman's marriage is rocky, such an experience can push her and her husband to the edge; the final outcome could be separation and divorce. For those who have this occur, it is not that*

your husband left you because your breast is gone. It is because of a series of misfortunes and differences of opinions that have been further complicated by breast surgery. My personal opinion on this subject is: Good riddance to him. You deserved better all along.

Question: How are your parents doing emotionally since all of this happened?
Answer: They are doing well. Our family has always been close, but now we are even closer that we were before. They are both very active in volunteer work regarding raising funds to support cancer screening, education, awareness, and research, with a special focus on helping people in the community where they live.

Question: How is your daughter?
Answer: She couldn't be better. She has been one of my best supporters and has educated other teenagers like herself about my experience. (She also is no longer worried about being small-breasted, having graduated in the summer of '94 into a 34 D bra!) I am constantly amazed at how resilient children can be; if we listen closely to what they have to say, we too can benefit from their wisdom. You will find that a five-year-old granddaughter looking at her grandmother soaking in the tub is perfectly accepting of her appearance and is completely unconcerned about the fact that she has one breast instead of two. That's because children know what unconditional love is.

Question: In what other ways do you consider having breast cancer a positive experience?
Answer: I have met people who, under normal circumstances, I would never have met. I have been

given the opportunity to spend time with breast cancer survivors who became club members after me and help them through the difficult moments that can only be shared and conquered with the help of another club member. I have felt the exhilaration of being present for the Susan G. Komen Race for the Cure Breast Cancer events where you are physically surrounded by thousands of other club members and their supporters. I have been given the opportunity to speak to large audiences as well as small groups such as breast cancer support groups, whose volunteers work with cancer patients and organizations holding fundraisers for cancer research and awareness. With each presentation, I feel rejuvenated just as if I were an Energizer bunny.

Question: Did you decide to name your other prosthesis after your second mastectomy?
Answer: Yes! Betty's roommate is named Bobbie. (Bobbie Sue to be precise.)

Question: Do you think that you will always do volunteer work for the Reach to Recovery Program?
Answer: Yes. I certainly hope so. And I want to see that program continue to evolve to meet the special needs of women with breast cancer. With with hospitalization length of stay averaging only one day, we need to develop additional mechanisms to support breast cancer patients after surgery. One of the things that I have noticed about the new club members whom I visit at the hospital is their sense of bonding with me, particularly once I tell them that I have opted not to have reconstruction done. They look at my chest and smile. They aren't smiling because they want to be socially polite to Betty and Bobbie Sue; they smile, I think, because they realize that I am an equal on the same playing field as they are on. I am a walking example that there is life, love,

joy, and happiness after breast cancer and that reconstruction isn't a requirement to achieve that happiness—it is an option.

Question: Where do you see cancer research going now?
Answer: We are on the brink of a new era of research methodology. In the past, treatments for cancer have focused their approach on what Dr. Susan Love calls the slash, poison, and burn methods. Slash—cut out the cancer. Poison—use chemotherapy to destroy it. Burn—use radiation to kill it. Now we are entering a biological era—gene identification, antibody therapy, vaccines. Rather than using the traditional ways of treating cancer, scientists are looking at developing ways to help the body repair its own cells that have mutated and will eventually turn into cancer cells. (Few people realize that a cancer cell is one of your own cells that has mutated and "gone bad.")

Question: What role do you want to play in the future regarding breast cancer treatment?
Answer: I want to be and stay wherever the action is. I want to help organizations that are committed to prevention. I want to be involved with researchers who are developing ways to provide early detection for premenopausal women, since so often conventional mammography doesn't pick up all tiny tumors, especially for women under age forty. I want to facilitate ways in which the care and treatment that are provided to women with breast cancer are the best, meeting patients' expectations regarding physical, psychological, cultural, and spiritual needs. One group of people often left to fend for themselves emotionally are the mothers of women with breast cancer. My mother and I are starting a support group for them. It is called Mothers Supporting Daughters

with Breast Cancer. It is a devastating experience for a mother to see her daughter go through such an experience. Many mothers carry guilt if they too have had breast cancer. Other mothers who have not been touched by this villain themselves wish that it was happening to them rather than to their daughter. These women need special support from one another and from others who have weathered the storm ahead of them. Mr. Greenberg, from the Jodee Institute, shares my commitment to develop such a program for these women. Having a clinical background, being a breast cancer survivor, and having expertise in the field of quality of care measurements, I am in a unique situation; hopefully I can offer a lot to those organizations looking to improve the quality of care and services provided to women with breast cancer and their families.

I have a postcard that I purchased for myself as a reminder of how women are viewed in society. It is a photograph of a young girl, about age ten, who is standing on the beach with a woman about thirty years of age. This woman is probably her mother, but she could also be an aunt or a neighbor or even an older sister. They are both wearing T-shirts and have their eyes closed as they stand with their chests proudly sticking out as they arch their necks back and drink in all of the sunshine, surf, and salt air. The T-shirt on the child says, "Watch this space." This photo means so many things to me: the realization of how important breasts are in our society; the realization that every girl wants to "watch her space" grow normally and still be attached to them when she dies of old age.

I am a believer in fate. I think that things happen to us for a reason. Two years ago I didn't really know just how precious life is. That's because I wasn't aware of my own mortality. Having looked the Grim Reaper in the face and having seen him smile at me, I now value each day. The sunset is gorgeous even if it is raining.

There are those who *say* that they want to help in the fight against breast cancer and there are those who *do something* to help with the fight. We need to encourage and facilitate more watchers to be doers. I am a doer. I want to see more doers. If you are a watcher, please become a doer. If you are already a doer, thank you. I'll be watching for you at breast cancer rallies, researcher conferences, support group meetings, and health fairs. As a united force with enough doers, we can prevent breast cancer.

Chapter 19
The Parents' Chapter

Dad's Section

It was rather strange last evening when my daughter Lillie called and asked me if I would write a little bit about being a parent of a cancer victim. Since I consider myself a rough and tough farmer, it is very difficult to say the things that I feel, or to put them into print, but if you are the unfortunate person who has been diagnosed as having cancer, bear with me and share my thoughts for a few minutes.

I was watching a program on the TV when our daughter called, and I borrow the title from that program: *The Day the Bubble Burst.* That was the story of the 1929 market crash. Having started out as very poor farmers and struggled to make ends meet, we finally broke through; I thought we had it all. We had political power, prestige in the community, and the financial ability to buy the things we needed, or at least anything we thought we needed.

On the beginning of the day the bubble burst I was in the shop some one hundred feet away from the house when I heard a noise. I went into the house thinking that my wife was laughing; it is very unusual for her to really break up.

When I found her on the sofa, I realized that she really was more than broken up. She had broken down, I think, for the first time in her whole life. Finally, I got her quieted down enough to hear Lillie's news that she had cancer. Had I contributed to it? Many other things came to mind. Why my family? Why my child? Why not me? When I crawled back in my big, green, glass-enclosed monster, where I was by myself on a farm tractor, I had a lot of time to think. How when she was a child growing up that she was fortunate, or unfortunate, perhaps, to be born to two workaholic parents. I did not take the time when she was growing up to be with her as I should have. I was busy keeping the wolf from the door and attempting to make a comfortable future for us.

Lillie was very subtle in knowing how to get what she wanted. She worked for what she wanted and needed. I remember that our house was a rather rough-looking old farmhouse when she was growing up. Her subtle way of waking me up was to go out in the yard and use her talents as an artist to paint the farmhouse where we live. When I saw the house in a picture I knew then it was time to fix up the place. I fixed up the outbuildings and I bought new machinery, so I guess I went on a binge to rebuild the house and to make things look better around here. But this was her way to get what she needed and what she knew her mother wanted.

Lillie touched many people when she was growing up. When I once had a serious chemical burn, she would drive fifty miles one way after being in class all day to give my injury a Betadine scrub so that my leg would not get infected and carry scars. She worked for Dr. Kaufman in Rock Hall for a brief time when she finished nursing school. Since then I have heard many people remark that she was incredibly compassionate. They said that they couldn't have made it without her. Compassion has been her trademark. Doing for others and not asking for anything in return. You ask why cancer occurs in this type of person? Not being a religious person, it is difficult to say the things that you would like to say, but perhaps by her having cancer she will be able to educate and help many, many others, including parents and children.

When you hear the word cancer of your daughter and you have a beautiful granddaughter coming of age, your thoughts leave the other members of your family and go to the daughter and granddaughter. You wonder who will raise the girl if her mother dies. Where will she go to school? What will she miss out on? After a day of thinking about these things, I was able to say to my wife, in full belief, "Don't worry. Lil will make it." Since the beginning of this crisis I felt Lil would see her child raised and educated. Now, a year later, we know that she will.

As a father, I have gone back over the farm activities we had while our children were growing up. We knew nothing about the chemicals we used on the farms. The spittle bug on the hay we sprayed with a chemical. The flies in the barn we sprayed with DDT. There were no restrictions or guidance. We thought that if a little would work, we'd put on more. The airplanes flew the cornfields with Toxiphene and other related chemicals for cutworm. We handled chemicals of all kinds on the farm that were used in the production of corn, soybeans, hay, and cattle. I looked back, wondering if some of these were the culprit. We lived across from Aberdeen and Edgewood, which were proving grounds for chemicals. Did this cause her cancer? When she was a child, did the ships coming down the bay, pumping out their bilges, contribute to it? Perhaps it was Mother Nature and God saying, "Well, we need to wake up some people really bad and have them realize the dangers in the environment." I think I can say without contradiction that Lillie's experiences changed our lives.

I know that Lillie is one of the most compassionate people I have ever known, but if there could be a way to be more compassionate, I think this has made her even more so. Personally, as her father, I've always felt that her hand on my shoulder or her standing by my bed when I'm ill has a tranquilizing effect equal to any medicine. She and I have a close relationship. When we see each other, we either hold hands or put our arms around each other and it is not necessary to say anything. We know what each other is thinking.

As I look back at her position, discovering that she had cancer, I realized that maybe something made her set her life up. She had a good husband, a good job, and many friends, and I think this was her salvation. The friends she had made here as well as in other places seemed to unite in prayer and in best wishes. I suppose that if I had to sum the source of her recovery up, prayer played one of the biggest roles, but her laughter and happiness that she displayed to other people in hiding her own fears had to be. Lillie knows how to laugh; she knows how to enjoy life; she knows how to be compassionate with other people. These things have been her salvation.

If you are unfortunate enough to be the recipient of the news that you have the dreaded cancer, don't try to blame yourself; don't try to blame everyone else; don't ask why you got cancer. If any advice could be given, it is this: Take a big yellow pad. Put down the good things that have happened in your life, then put down the bad. You will probably find out that the good things outweigh the others. If you know a victim, be there when you are needed and have the good sense to let the person have time to herself when you are not needed. Realize that you take life one day at a time and that money won't buy everything—that friends, prayers, memories of good times, good laughter, and a close relationship with your family will probably help the doctors and the hospitals to restore you to good health.

Mom's Section

There was a song written many decades ago that indicated that it wasn't important how much you had; the importance was what you did with what you had. Those words could have been said about us. In 1946, when we were married, we had little money and dreams of better things and, fortunately, the energy to attempt to make some of the dreams pan out.

God had blessed us with two "whole" children who brought us tremendous amounts of joy. They were a month short of three years apart, spacing which some of our friends indicated was the worst thing that could happen. Well, we proved them wrong on that score and on many others. It turned out, in my mind, anyway, to be perfect timing. The older one, our son, thought it was wonderful to have a little sister. And, being a take-charge type, he apparently assigned himself as her protector.

As you learned in earlier chapters, our daughter seemed to be plagued with various ailments, yet always appeared to be the healthier child. Fortunately, none of the unusual happenings seemed to deter her from accomplishing fantastic things at very early ages. Being on a farm afforded both of our children on-the-scene education that takes years for city or town children to learn. This really gave them a leg up on some other students.

At the age of three, our daughter began performing before audiences, singing songs we learned together—songs that were long and difficult for many adults to learn. In this way, she never had stage fright or knew what being bashful meant. It was second nature, almost like breathing. I really believe that our music was the thread that bound the family together. We always felt the need to turn to it when things were going sour and it helped us see our way clear to survive the difficulty at hand.

There have been a number of times in my life when I have made the remark, "If I can get through this mess, I can live through anything." As I look back at some of the things that I termed "a crisis," it almost makes me laugh. Some of them were child's play by comparison to the things that were waiting around the corner in later years. It sort of reminds me of the progress that children show. In the early stages, learning to walk is the biggest thing in their lives. Later it might be the challenge of riding a two-wheeler. Sometimes it might be learning how to produce what the teacher expects, even though the child dislikes the format that he/she insists the term paper must comply with.

When our school board changed the district boundary lines for students who attended Chestertown High School and Rock Hall High School, making it necessary for our children to change schools, even though we had not moved, I was ready to throw up my hands, or my fists, and do battle. These had been rival schools ever since they were established. Our son was about to enter his senior year, so he was permitted to complete his last year in Chestertown, if we provided transportation; however, our daughter was entering the ninth grade, so there was no way for her to continue attending the Chestertown school. The two had worked out a wonderful plan earlier. He would play basketball and she would be a cheerleader. Now that he could drive, they could attend games together and come home in our car without making it necessary for us to transport them when they returned to the school grounds on the bus. They were crushed to learn that this would not happen.

So, my famous statement came forth: "If I can get through this mess, I can live through anything." The rival schools played the games on different nights, of course, except when they played each other. We would attend the home games and on one side for the first half and on the other side for the second half. I thought that was one of the most difficult times of my life, but I did not know what was waiting around the corner.

We survived. Many years have passed since the rival-school year and many other crises came into the picture. Each time I came forth with my famous statement and each time I wondered if I would be conditioned for the next challenge that had my name on it. I began to be able to adjust better, or at least I thought I could. Many times folks did not understand that my ability to cope with these crushing blows was not insensitivity, but strength to see a situation through to the end without folding. It was holding on in spite of adversity.

We have had hail storms that destroyed corn crops, fires that wiped us out of the dairy business, and droughts that made us wonder why we put so much blood, sweat, and tears into the farming business. All of these things seemed to swat us down, but we came back to do battle another day. These situations make one feel somewhat helpless, but the hope of doing better the next time is never destroyed.

My husband's mother once said that when a child is born, a mother worries about it until either she or it dies. She was probably correct in making that statement. I thought I could handle nearly anything that came my way. Through levelheadedness and prayer, many of the things that came my way were overcome. Then we had the word from our daughter—this delightful, bubbly young woman with wit so sharp that one wondered why she did not have a daily newspaper column or some other way to share it with others who need to have a laugh to survive the day. When I heard her say that she was going for a mammogram, I knew that something was very wrong.

All of the articles I have read indicated that women should begin having mammograms performed when they turn forty. She was only thirty-eight, so she would not do this unless she thought there was need for it. Then she confessed that four years earlier she had one done because there was a cyst in her right breast. It was drained and everything was fine. How much more has gone on that she has not wanted to worry us with, was my comment to myself. Sure enough, the mammogram showed another cyst in the breast, but she was assured that it could be drained, as before. Then the film of the other breast was checked and there was something suspicious on it. This was the breast that had given no indication that anything was wrong.

The waiting period between the time we knew that something was suspicious and when the pathology report from the open biopsy was due was an eternity. Each day when she returned from work I would call to find out what she knew. Each day she still had heard nothing. I prayed that everything was all right. Finally, on this day when I called, there was a hesitation about what she knew. Then she quietly said, "It wasn't what we wanted." Then I knew this was a new crisis. I contained my composure until I hung up the phone.

At that moment I felt as though someone had just told me that she was dead and that I should prepare for a funeral in two days. I know that sounds very strange, particularly from a person who has always been able to hold together regardless of what was going on. But this time I felt that the wrong generation had been attacked. It was *not* her turn. I could handle this much better myself. Mothers can heal themselves easier than they can handle their loved ones being in pain.

I began crying and sobbing, as I said before, as though she were already gone. What am I going to do to help her now? I thought. How am I going to help our granddaughter? How am I going to help our son-in-law? And, worst of all, how am I going to help my husband, her father, who believes that she can almost walk on water? When my husband came into the house and found me weeping, he surmised what was wrong. All I had to say was that I had heard from Lillie. He later said that it was the first time in the fifty years that we had known each other that he saw me go to pieces immediately upon hearing bad news. Usually I held up until a crisis was over before I showed any affect at all.

"I can't stand it," I repeated again and again. "There is nothing fair about this. She doesn't smoke or drink. All that she is guilty of is working too hard. Why are energetic people punished like this? I could handle this much easier if it happened to me." I went on and on. He tried to comfort me, but there was little he could do when he felt as bad as I did. It is the most helpless feeling that one can experience: Your child is notified that she has cancer and there is no magic wand to make it disappear. It isn't just a bad dream that you will come out of, either. There is no way to escape.

There were several things that I was working on at that time, and I was making notes about them, I was constantly using the wrong date. I was hung up in May, it seemed. That was prior to the announcement that cancer had found another fertile spot to have fun. I suppose I wanted time to reverse, so it would not be known that we had a new crisis. One's brain works in strange ways. I completely forgot my sister's wedding anniversary and her husband's birthday. They came and went in July, but I was still catching myself dating things May.

Nothing seemed to be going right for me. Fortunately I did not have what I used to call "a real job" away from home. All of the work I did was free-lance or keeping the farm books, so my use of the wrong month could be corrected without harm. I functioned much like a robot. Many things were done by rote. Many other things were not done at all. Some things that had seemed very important no longer had meaning or value. I called all of my friends in various churches and asked that our daughter be placed on their prayer list. We had people praying in the entire county, many other parts of Maryland, in the District of Columbia, in Colorado, and halfway around the world (since our son and his family were stationed in Japan).

After the mastectomy was completed, there was another waiting period. I was not doing well in the section marked "patience." I felt as though I wanted to find the persons in the labs where the testing was being done and make sure they were doing their job properly. The family accuses me of wanting to have things done properly anyway. Why not? That's what a person is paid to do. I also wanted the folks in the labs to get moving before I was totally crazed with concern about the whole thing. Fortunately I was not denying that this was serious, even though I wanted the clock to reverse to a time when everyone was well, or at least when we thought we were. I just wanted answers and I wanted them pronto, not later.

As the days dragged on, friends inquired about our daughter each time I happened to meet them, on the street, in the grocery store, anywhere. Each time I found myself being teary-eyed and had to apologize for showing such emotion. One day, however, when a family acquaintance asked about her, tears welled up in my eyes as I told him. He quickly said, "Oh, I'm sorry that I asked. Please excuse me." I knew then that I had to get hold of myself. The last thing that I wanted was to turn off folks who were genuinely interested, so I had a firm talk with myself and made it very clear that I could do better. As luck would have it, I saw the same man that evening at a meeting and went to him to thank him for making me realize that I could control my inner feelings, particularly when folks who inquire are inquiring about her health.

Fortunately, the lymph nodes were negative, so we felt that the tide finally had turned in our favor. Now it was really time to give thanks for blessings. God has spared all of us for a reason, I believe. We now need to continue to be crusaders who tell others that there is life after cancer; that there is life after mastectomy; that parents can be supportive to each other as well as to the family member who is the cancer survivor. Now I can say that Lillie has opted to lose a body part in order to save her life. She has taught all of us many lessons through the years, but making us realize how precious life can be is probably the most important lesson of all.

Chapter 20

Helpful Hints for Breast Cancer Patients, their Families, and Concerned Friends

This chapter is designed to be a resource for women who have been diagnosed with breast cancer. It contains information for the patient, as well as suggestions for family members and friends who will be involved in her treatment and recovery. Based on your individual situation, you may choose not to utilize all of the sections of this chapter. It is merely here as a reference for you.

Helping her to retain her femininity and womanliness:

When a woman is confronted with the news that she is going to lose her breasts, it is not uncommon that, accompanying the feelings of fear of death from cancer, she feels fear of losing her femininity. Breasts have long been a symbol of womanhood. The loss of a breast can cause a woman to doubt her attractiveness and make her fear that she will be considered less of a woman. Below are some suggestions for small gifts that can help to enhance her womanliness and promote a more positive self-image. For those of you who are on a tight budget, these items can be purchased in most Cosmetic Centers, Rite Aid Pharmacies, Crabtree and Evelyn Caldor, and other similar chain stores at very reasonable prices. Your Avon representative is also an excellent person to contact to purchase these items as well. It is particularly nice to purchase small containers of these items. You might consider the "one-time use" samplers that usually cost less than a dollar. Items such as the facial mask come in a flat, one-time–use pouch and can be mailed in an envelope with a greeting card. Items that are inexpensive and can be mailed in an envelope accompanied by a card or personal note are indicated with an asterisk (*).

Bubble bath (sizes range from tiny travel-sized plastic bottles to jumbo economy size).

* Facial mask (a favorite is the new antistress masks).

* Sachets for her lingerie drawer (some come in flat envelopes; others are in satin or mesh netting).

Fragranced soaps.

Small, soft pillows (for use after surgery to support her affected arm).

Book of verses about womanhood or the special friendship shared among women.

* Bookmark. (These can be especially fun! They range from inspirational to having photos of naked men on them. You can write a special note on the back of them to her as well.)

Jewelry (a small locket or perhaps a charm for a charm bracelet or necklace).

Romance novels.

* A gift certificate for a facial.

* A gift certificate for a makeover.

* A gift certificate for a trip to the beauty parlor to have her hair done.

* A gift certificate for a manicure or pedicure.

Nightgown. (One size fits all, opened down the front. These are available in Sears and other stores that carry fuller women's clothes. Even if the individual is not a fuller size, it is smart to have this kind of gown for the post-op period. Choose a pretty pastel color.)

Flowers with a special card that tells her how special she is and how much she is loved.

* A gift certificate for a romantic dinner with the man that she loves. (If this gift is from the man, then perhaps just a card with a date and time you plan to pick her up; tell her where you'll be taking her.)

* A gift certificate for an overnight stay for two in a hotel that has Jacuzzis in the rooms.

Information that the breast cancer patient will benefit from:
(Remember, with knowledge there is personal empowerment.)

The Cancer Information Center
By telephone: (toll-free) 1-800-4-CANCER
These numbers are assessable from 9 A.M. to 10 P.M.
Alaska: 1-800-638-6070 on weekdays
    and from 10 A.M. until 6 P.M. on Sat.
Hawaii: 1-800-524-1234

They can be reached by mail at:

Office of Cancer Communications
National Cancer Institute
Besthesda, Maryland 20692

The Cancer Information Center will provide you information about the newest treatment for breast cancer as well as send you literature in the mail about diagnosis and treatment.

Pamphlets that the American Cancer information center can provide free of charge:

Adjuvant Therapy—Facts for Women with Breast Cancer
Advanced Cancer: Living Each Day
Answers to Questions about Metastatic Cancer
Breast Biopsy: What You Should Know
Breast Exams: What You Should Know
Breast Cancer: Treatment Options
Breast Reconstruction: A Matter of Choice
Chemotherapy and You
Eating Hints: Resource for the Diet and Nutrition During Cancer Treatment
Mastectomy: A Treatment for Breast Cancer
Questions and Answers about Breast Lumps
Questions and Answers about Pain Control
Radiation Therapy and You
Taking Time: Support for the People with Cancer and the People Who Care about Them
What You Need to Know About Breast Cancer
When Cancer Recurs: Meeting the Challenge Again
A Patient's Guide to Understanding Novaldex (Tamoxifen)
After Breast Cancer—A Guide to Follow-up
Komen Foundation Post Mastectomy Self-Examination
Questions to Ask Your Doctor About Swelling of the Arm

American Cancer Society
90 Park Avenue
New York, NY 10016

(212) 599-8200
1-800-ACS-2345

The American Cancer Society will send you information on treatment, detection, prevention, as well as local services available in your own area. They offer three specific programs for breast cancer patients.

Reach to Recovery is a program operated by volunteers who have had mastectomies. They provide emotional support and helpful hints to women who have had a mastectomy or are about to undergo such a procedure. They usually come to the hospital to see the patient shortly after the surgery has been done. This program is usually initiated by the patient's doctor, but it is wise to request it yourself.

CanSurmount and **I Can Cope** are general programs also offered by this organization to unite volunteers, patients with cancer (as well as their families), and health care professionals to provide educational and emotional support.

Y-ME
National Organization For Breast Cancer Support
National Hotline 1-800-221-2141

This organization provides emotional support and information about breast cancer treatment. It is staffed by volunteers who are breast cancer survivors.

Mothers Supporting Daughters with Breast Cancer
c/o Charmayne Dierker
21710 Bayshore Road
Chesterton, MD 21620
(410) 728-1982

This is a newly formed, nonprofit organization dedicated to helping mothers cope with the emotional impact breast cancer has on themselves and their daughters. It was founded in 1995 and was developed by my mother and I. We are eager to make it a national organization too. Please write for more information. We're here to help and also are seeking more mothers to work as volunteers nationwide.

Look Good . . . Feel Better
1-800-395-LOOK

Developed by Cosmetic, Toiletry, and Fragrance Association, in cooperation with ACS to help patients undergoing cancer treatment to improve their appearance. The National Cosmetology Association also participates in this program.

Dr. Susan Love's Breast Book
by Susan Love, M.D., 1990
Addison Wesley Publishing Company

This is an excellent book that includes drawings and descriptions of answers to nearly every question a woman or her family may have about breast disease, with a ninety-percent focus on breast cancer.

The Informed Woman's Guide To Breast Health
by Kerry Anne McGinn, RN
Bull Publishing Company

Breast Cancer Action
1280 Columbia Avenue #204
San Francisco, CA 94133
(415) 922-8279

Breast Cancer Action is a grass-roots organization made up of breast cancer survivors and their supporters. They actively promote increased awareness about breast cancer and strive to encourage efforts to prevent and eventually cure breast cancer. Newsletters are published bimonthly for a nominal annual fee. The newsletters are full of current information about breast cancer research, the status of various legislative bills under discussion that would benefit breast cancer prevention, and news about breast cancer awareness programs held in regional areas.

National Alliance of Breast Cancer Organizations
1180 Ave of the Americas
2nd Floor
New York, NY 10036
(212) 719-0154

The Susan G. Komen Breast Cancer Foundation

A national race for the CureTM is held annually in many cities to provide funds for breast cancer research, education, and treatment. For information about breast health or breast cancer, call the Komen Foundation's help line at 1-800-IM-AWARE.

CANCERVIVE INC.
6500 Wilshire Boulevard
Suite 500
Los Angeles, CA 90048
(310) 203-9232

Cancervive Inc. assists cancer survivors to face and overcome the challenges of life after cancer.

My Image After Breast Cancer
(703) 461-9595

My Image After Breast Cancer provides a magazine devoted to research and the latest treatment in breast cancer for a nominal fee.

National Breast Cancer Coalition
P. O. Box 66373
Washington, DC 20035

Formed in 1991 with more than one hundred forty organizations, representing several million patients, professionals, women, their families and friends, NBCC has had a significant impact on general awareness about the breast cancer epidemic and a major influence on public policy.

Prodigy Service
445 Hamilton Ave
White Plains, NY 10601
(914) 933-8000

America Online
8619 Westwood Center Drive
Vienna, VA 22182-2285
1-800-827-3338

Both companies offer a computer software package that provides a wide variety of services via modem. One of their less-advertised features is a breast cancer medical support group. Via your computer, you can ask questions of other breast cancer victims and survivors and receive as well as provide to others emotional support and helpful hints about their experiences with surgery, radiation therapy, chemotherapy, etc. You also get literature about cancer research being done worldwide.

The Wellness Community
Dulaney Center II
Dulaney Valley Road
Baltimore, MD 21204
(410) 832-2719

Founded by Harold H. Benjamin, Ph.D., who became interested in the psychosocial aspects of cancer-patient care after his wife developed breast cancer. The first program opened June 1982 in Santa Monica, California. Now there are facilities across the United States. The primary purpose of the program is to help as many cancer patients as possible recover to the greatest extent possible by providing a free program of psychosocial support in which cancer patients learn to actively fight for their recovery along with their physicians and health teams.

Their various programs include free psychotherapy sessions, group discussions, education sessions, family support groups, relaxation sessions, nutrition help, exercise, social events, and special networking groups (one of which is exclusively for breast cancer patients). In the Baltimore area they can be located at the address/phone listed above.

Local Chapter of your American Cancer Society
Yellow Pages

Call your local ACS chapter to receive literature about breast cancer support groups in your area.

Mastectomy Supply Stores: Yes! Sometimes these stores have sales on mastectomy bras! It's smart to call them around Memorial Day and Labor Day for the best buys on mastectomy swimwear too.

Wig Stores: If you are anticipating chemotherapy and the drugs to be used usually cause hair loss, it is recommended to be fitted for a wig before you start your therapy. These stores often carry pamphlets on creative ways to wear scarves on you head as well.

Jodee's Bra Inc.
3100 North 20th Avenue
Hollywood, FL 33020
Shop Toll Free: 1-800-821-2767

This is a company that has truly pioneered the mastectomy bra business. They carry a wide variety of mastectomy bras, prostheses, and other accessories that help provide a balanced and comfortable fit. Their mail-order catalog is sent to you quarterly and often offers sales! They also carry swimsuits and lingerie, specially designed for a woman's needs after breast surgery, whether that be a mastectomy or lumpectomy.

Their fitters are trained to ensure a proper fit, recognizing from this company's experience over the last two decades that many problems that women have, including some orthopedic and neurological problems, are due to poor fittings and lack of information regarding what to look for in a good prosthesis and bra fitting. It has been felt to be the most closeted aspect to breast surgery post-op. A proper fitting by a qualified fitter can help prevent neck and back problems that can result from an improper fit.

The loss of a breast causes an imbalance to the body, therefore it is important to restore balance to the body by wearing a weighted breast form. There are specific checkpoints that Jodee recommends always be considered when being fitted. Jodee bras meet all of these checkpoint standards. However, if you are purchasing a bra from another company or local mastectomy supply store that doesn't carry Jodee products, it is smart to follow Jodee's well-established criterion.

Jodee emphasizes that "a breast form is only as effective as the bra that carries it." They are right. They have in their catalog a pictorial guide that explains in simple and clearly defined terms the checkpoints on a bra that must be met to ensure a perfect fit. It would be worth your while to call their toll-free number and get a catalog so that you have this instruction guide available to you no matter where you are fitted. In my opinion, you will find their staff to be such compassionate people to deal with and their products of such high quality that you won't want to shop anywhere else.

Their president emphasizes the importance of maintaining a woman's privacy. Dealing through such a mail-order catalog fulfills this personal need while simultaneously meeting your other physical and psychological needs.

Louise Rose, vice-president of Jodee and a national consultant says, "Every woman needs to know what to look for in a good fitting, for she fits herself every day. Where she goes to a store to be fitted, she should have in hand the following listed checkpoints to assure a good fitting because not all fitters are equal in their training and experience."

The checkpoints that are recommended are listed below:

1. Does your bra touch the center breast bone? Good separation prevents "peekout."

2. Does your bra ride up? Wear it snug, not loose, so the bandeau can work.

3. Does your breast form (prosthesis) feel heavy? Adjust straps so the breast form is close to your body.

4. Does the breast form projection match your natural side? Try smaller or larger breast forms.

5. Are you wearing straps close to your neck to prevent grabbing and creating tilted shoulders? (A common cause of shoulder and neck pain.)

6. Is there a depressed area above the breast form? Sew in a form tab to fill this cavity. (These tabs are available in the Jodee catalog. I, Lillie Shockney, haven't seen them available elsewhere.)

7. Does your bra pull or twist to the side? Reasons for this can be:
    a) Cup form too small on natural side.
    b) Breast form too light in weight.
    c) Flesh out from underarm causes bra to twist or slide. Use foam cushion to fill in this area. (These cushions are very hard to find but are available through Jodee.)

Land's End, Inc.
1 Land's End Lane
Dodgeville, WI 53595
1-800-356-4444

Land's End carries bathing suits that have a shelf bra in them which can be easily converted into a pocket for use with a breast prosthesis. It isn't advertised, though, as a mastectomy bathing suit usually is. The arm area nicely covers up the incisional area and the sculptured neckline is slightly higher than standard, thus providing you all the concealment you need. Their tank tops are great for concealing the axillary incision as well. And they wear extremely well!

B & B Breast Prosthesis Company
P. O. Box 5731
2417 Bank Drive, Suite 201
Boise, ID 83705
1-800-262-2789 or (208) 343-9696

B & B has a special prosthesis designed by a breast cancer survivor as an alternative to heavier silicone breast forms. It fits in a regular bra and is made of nylon and cotton and cushioned with fiberfill. It's washable and costs around seventy dollars including shipping.

Information that is valuable to the husband/significant sweetie:

The woman you love isn't going through this medical crisis alone. You, too, feel the emotional pain and anxiety along with her. It is a time to show her that you will stick behind her. It is a time to let her see that your love for her does not exist in her flesh that she is about to lose. Though it is a hard thing to ask of anyone, this is a time to demonstrate your strength. She needs to rely on you to help her in making personal decisions about treatment options. She also needs you to carry the load when it comes to her immediate post-op recovery at home. The following books might be helpful to you as you proceed down your mate's path of transformation from breast cancer victim to breast cancer survivor:

Man to Man: When the Woman You Love Has Breast Cancer
by Andy Murcia and Bob Stewart, 1989
St. Martin's Press, New York

This is a marvelous book written by Ann Jillian's husband and a close friend of theirs who also had a wife diagnosed with breast cancer during same time that Ann did. It is written for men. I personally found the book to be excellent and wished that I had known about the book during my diagnostic and treatment phase. You may need to order it from a book store because I have found that not many stores keep a ready supply in stock. Walden Books and BDalton can order it in quickly though (about seven days).

Dr. Susan Love's Breast Book

This book is referenced above and is worth the time for you, too, to read it as well. The drawings will give you a sense of what to expect post-op, though the drawings are subtle.

**Call her breast surgeon or family doctor
for a private phone consultation.**

Her physician may be able to connect you with another husband who has weathered the storm of breast cancer in the recent past. There is a real sense of relief to be able to talk to someone who has been there and made it through. If her physician is not helpful, the Reach to Recovery Program might be.

Talk with your clergymen.

Oftentimes, we don't turn to those who are standing ready, willing, and able to help us. Prayer is a powerful tool in the fight against cancer. Your church may also have support group meetings for members who are also going through the trials and tribulations of such a disease. Remember, there is also power in numbers.

Plan ahead. Make a schedule of the things that must be done before, during, and after her surgery.

Women are notorious for worrying about things, so spare her the additional stress of worrying about paying bills, finding sitters to watch the kids while she's in the hospital, etc. Sit down and make out a plan. She can help you if she insists. Recruit family and friends to help out with child care, dog care, fixing meals, et cetera. By doing so, she can concentrate on getting well and not on family crisis management. Everyone will sleep better for it.

Spend time alone, just the two of you.

She needs to feel your strength and love. Time to talk about what she feels and is most worried about is important time to spend. All too often we are all living in the fast lane with no real quality time to spend together. If ever there was a time to rearrange priorities, this is it. Put her first. Share your concerns. Most importantly, share your love.

Write down questions you both have to take with you to your doctor's appointments. It's too easy to forget once you are there and your adrenaline is pumping.

A handy place is usually in a small notebook that will fit in your pocket. Keep it with you all the time so that it isn't forgotten on appointment days. Also, record what the doctor tells you at each appointment. When nerves are frazzled, memories can also be a bit blurry.

Above all else, THINK POSITIVE!

If ever there is someone who must remain optimistic, it is you! Breast cancer can be beat! Surgery, radiation, and chemotherapy are only a part of the treatment. Your optimism and unrelenting love is the other part. If you're feeling down, see someone that you trust to talk to and confide in. You are a very valuable player in the healing process. Watch the newspaper for special breast cancer education programs held at shopping malls, local hospitals, and cancer support organizations like The Wellness Community. Get involved with these types of programs so that you can learn more as well as get to meet other club members and club-member supporters.

DOs and DON'Ts for the woman about to undergo a mastectomy:

First the DOs:
DO take time to get all of your questions answered by your physician. You deserve the answers; he owes you the time. Make a list of your questions and take the list with you when you have your next appointment.

DO purchase a large (one size fits most/all) nightgown that buttons or snaps down the front. You will be much more comfortable in it than your regular nightgowns when you first come home from your mastectomy surgery. These gowns have large arm holes and are very flowing. There is room for you, your bandages, and your drainage tubes.

DO stock up on some basic dressing supplies, such as a small box of four-by-four gauze pads and a roll of paper or adhesive tape. Though the hospital will send some home with you, it usually isn't enough.

DO let family and friends help you. This is not the time to be a martyr. Let neighbors feed the dog (and kids for that matter) while you are in the hospital. Casseroles are always welcome! Let your sister vacuum for you after you are home recovering. Your recovery will go smoother and faster if you take the time to take care of yourself.

DO switch your wrist watch from one wrist to another if you are having a mastectomy on the side that you usually wear your watch. It is not advisable to wear anything constricting on the arm that coincides with your surgery. This is because some or all of your lymph nodes will be removed. These glands carry fluid away from your upper extremity and help to ward off infection. Maintaining good circulation is promoted by avoiding constricting objects such as watches, tight-fitting rings, and tight, elastic sleeves.

DO share your thoughts and concerns with your spouse, other pertinent family members, and close friends. There is no reason to bear this burden alone. You'll feel better, and so will they.

DO get fitted for a wig in advance of starting your chemotherapy treatments (if this is to be part of your adjuvant therapy). The fit will be better and as a result you will be happier with your appearance. Just remember, when your hair grows back, it will be healthier, fuller, and have more body than ever before. You'll never have another bad-hair day again!

DO stay active. Enjoy whatever activities you previously did that are within reason during your surgical and adjuvant treatment. This is *not* the time to hibernate and close the walls in on your social life. Once your incision is well-healed and you have your doctor's permission, you might find it useful to use Summer's Eve feminine powder in your mastectomy bra to help reduce sweating during warm months or during active aerobic moments.

DO pamper yourself. This is a very appropriate time for long luxurious bubble baths, a trip to the sauna, a facial, and the purchase of that new fragrance of perfume that you've been wanting. I don't mean to imply that this is the time to spend your paycheck on frivolous things, but a ten-dollar manicure can go a long way to lifting your spirits on a day that is riddled with unpleasantries like receiving your chemotherapy appointment schedule.

DO talk with your clergy and other religious members close to you to gain additional support during these trying times ahead. Placing your faith in God will help you to restore your mind to a sense of peace.

Now for the DON'Ts:

DON'T give all of your bras away. You may be able to have them altered by having a pocket sewn in them to hold your breast prosthesis. Check with the stores that sell prostheses; they frequently have women who spend their entire day altering bras! They frequently don't advertise it, though.

DON'T give away your swimsuits either! Most suits are very easy to have pockets sewn in them. It would be a shame to toss your favorite floral suit away because you assume that you won't be able to wear it again after surgery. Even if it's cut low, you can have what is nicknamed a "privacy panel" sewn in it. This is a piece of cloth that matches the color/pattern of your suit and covers the upper portion of your swimsuit where your cleavage used to be. They work very well.

DON'T lose your sense of humor. Remember, it is one or your best weapons against cancer.